SPORTS AND ATHLETICS DEVELOPMENTS

SPORTS AND ATHLETICS DEVELOPMENTS

JAMES H. HUMPHREY
EDITOR

Nova Science Publishers, Inc.
New York

For permission to use material from this book please contact us:
Telephone 631-231-7269; Fax 631-231-8175
Web Site: http://www.novapublishers.com

NOTICE TO THE READER

The Publisher has taken reasonable care in the preparation of this book, but makes no expressed or implied warranty of any kind and assumes no responsibility for any errors or omissions. No liability is assumed for incidental or consequential damages in connection with or arising out of information contained in this book. The Publisher shall not be liable for any special, consequential, or exemplary damages resulting, in whole or in part, from the readers' use of, or reliance upon, this material. Any parts of this book based on government reports are so indicated and copyright is claimed for those parts to the extent applicable to compilations of such works.

Independent verification should be sought for any data, advice or recommendations contained in this book. In addition, no responsibility is assumed by the publisher for any injury and/or damage to persons or property arising from any methods, products, instructions, ideas or otherwise contained in this publication.

This publication is designed to provide accurate and authoritative information with regard to the subject matter covered herein. It is sold with the clear understanding that the Publisher is not engaged in rendering legal or any other professional services. If legal or any other expert assistance is required, the services of a competent person should be sought. FROM A DECLARATION OF PARTICIPANTS JOINTLY ADOPTED BY A COMMITTEE OF THE AMERICAN BAR ASSOCIATION AND A COMMITTEE OF PUBLISHERS.

LIBRARY OF CONGRESS CATALOGING-IN-PUBLICATION DATA
Available Upon Request

ISBN 978-1-60456-205-7

Published by Nova Science Publishers, Inc. ✤ New York

CONTENTS

PREFACE

Sports and athletics are at the focus of attention of millions and millions of people around the world - regardless of the level of the sport of athletic competition. There is perhaps more learned about life on the playing fields than anywhere else. Even the most disparate people can find common ground on sports or teams. This book brings together developments in this diverse field.

Chapter 1 - The purpose of this study was to examine the specific social conditions and contexts in which motor performance is facilitated or inhibited and to synthesize the findings of previous research into the theoretical framework that best explains the trends in the data. In 39 studies, the presence of others had small to moderate effects on motor performance. The main findings indicate that the mere presence of individuals does slightly facilitate performance. Similarly, in co-acting dyads, moderate facilitation effects were found for complex tasks. However, participating in activities with groups of individuals leads to decreased performance through social loafing. Evaluation also results in performance declines across all conditions. These meta-analytic results are discussed in relation to the Attentional Processes model.

Chapter 2 - We examined use of proactive (i.e., defensive) pessimism as a strategy employed by sport fans to assist them in coping with the possibility that their team will perform poorly. Proactive pessimism occurs as persons become more pessimistic about a self-relevant event as the event draws near. This suggests that fans may become more pessimistic about their team's chances of success as a season approaches. Use of this strategy was expected to be most prominent among fans with a high level of team identification for whom use of the strategy would be beneficial. However, these fans were not expected to lower their feelings of connection to the team as the season approached. Finally, we examined the potential impact of proactive pessimism on behavioral intentions (i.e., desire to attend the team's games). Participants completed a questionnaire packet four weeks prior to the start of the Major League Baseball season and then again one week prior. The packet assessed demographics, level of identification with one's favorite baseball team, and expectations for and excitement about the upcoming season. The results confirmed the expected pattern of effects as highly identified fans (but not those low in identification) reported lowered expectations at Time 2 relative to Time 1 (i.e., they became proactively pessimistic). Also as expected, there was no Time 1 to Time 2 change in connections to the team. Finally, the results indicated that lowly identified fans expressed greater interest in attending the team's games as the season approached while highly identified fans exhibited the opposite pattern.

Chapter 3 - The purpose of this study was to examine the relationships between the Desire to attend collegiate women's basketball (DES) and three aspects of attending collegiate women's basketball games. The participants were spectators of a National Collegiate Athletic Association (NCAA) Division I women's basketball game ranging in age from 18 to 70 ($N = 312$). The Modified Sports Consumers Questionnaire (Milne & McDonald, 1999) was administered during a basketball game. After exploratory factor analysis (EFA) and confirmatory factor analysis (CFA), three factors (Habit, Attitude, and Satisfaction) with 19 items were retained for Sports Spectator Behavior (SSB). Structural equation modeling was used to analyze the relationships among DES and three SSB factors. The findings revealed that the DES was positively related to the Habit of affiliating themselves with sports (HAB) and the Attitude toward watching sports (ATT), but negatively related to the Satisfaction of watching sports (SAT). The three main predictors of SSB account for 85% of the variance of DES.

Chapter 4 - The purpose of this study was to review previous prediction research in intercollegiate athletics, identify future trends in Division II Athletics, and compare predominately white colleges and universities (PWCU) to historically black colleges and universities (HBCU). Similar to previous research, this study utilized a modified Delphi technique to elicit responses from Athletic Directors and Senior Women Administrators of Division II level institutions. A total of 15 Athletic Directors and Senior Women Administrators responded to the first round of questionnaires and 29 in the second round. In all, 17 items were identified by the panelist in the areas of academics, NCAA governance, amateurism, gender equity, and financial conditions. The questionnaire further asked the respondents to indicate when the items may occur, the level of desirability of the item and impact that the item would have, and descriptive statistics were utilized to notate the average levels, and any anecdotal differences between HBCUs and PWCUs.

Chapter 5 - Recent burnout research has examined coaches and athletes collectively to determine the influence of coach behaviors on coach and athlete burnout. Results revealed a potential incongruity between decision-making behaviors and their influence on coach and athlete burnout. Therefore, the present study examined relationships between decision-making styles of coaches and burnout among coaches and athletes; gender influence on burnout was also examined. Collegiate swimmers and swimming coaches completed questionnaires assessing burnout and decision-making behaviors. Results revealed a significant relationship between athlete burnout and autocratic coaching behaviors. A significant inverse relationship emerged between athlete burnout and democratic behaviors. Significant main effects were found for democratic behaviors on exhaustion and depersonalization subscales; swimmers perceiving fewer democratic behaviors scored higher on these subscales. No significant relationships or gender differences were found with the coaches. Results suggest that coaches eliciting feedback from athletes could reduce the likelihood of burnout among those athletes without predisposing themselves.

Chapter 6 - The present study was designed to develop a 23-item scale to measure positive illusion in competitive athletes. Positive illusion is a multidimensional psychological construct consisting of the following 3 cognitive characteristics: self-aggrandizement, illusion of control, and unrealistic opitimism. Cronbach's alpha at .84 indicated relatively high internal consistency for the Positive Illusion Sport Scale. Convergent and discriminant validities were assessed by correlating scores from the Scale with scores of self-esteem, hopelessness, optimism, and depression. The Positive Illusion Sport Scale had a moderate positive correlation with self-esteem and optimism and a moderate negative correlation with hopelessness and depression. These findings demonstrate convergent and discriminant validity for the new instrument and suggest that it is psychometrically adequate for research and clinical purposes.

In: Sports and Athletics Developments
Editor: James H. Humphrey, pp. 1-28

Chapter 1

SOCIAL FACILITATION AND MOTOR/ATHLETIC PERFORMANCE: A META-ANALYSIS

*David P. Oviatt and Seppo E. Iso-Ahola**
University of Maryland
Department of Kinesiology

ABSTRACT

The purpose of this study was to examine the specific social conditions and contexts in which motor performance is facilitated or inhibited and to synthesize the findings of previous research into the theoretical framework that best explains the trends in the data. In 39 studies, the presence of others had small to moderate effects on motor performance. The main findings indicate that the mere presence of individuals does slightly facilitate performance. Similarly, in co-acting dyads, moderate facilitation effects were found for complex tasks. However, participating in activities with groups of individuals leads to decreased performance through social loafing. Evaluation also results in performance declines across all conditions. These meta-analytic results are discussed in relation to the Attentional Processes model.

* Correspondence to: Dr. Seppo Iso-Ahola, University of Maryland, Department of Kinesiology. College Park, MD 20742. Email: isoahol@umd.edu

Key words: Social influence, sports performance, mere presence, evaluation.

INTRODUCTION

Why is it that when faced with a pressured situation, in the company of others, some individuals prevail at their given task, while others seemingly choke and fail? Is it individual differences regarding past history and familiarity with such situations or tasks? Or, is there something about the mere presence of other individuals -- whether they are friends or strangers, supportive or critical? Rarely does the reply to such a broad question include one all-encompassing answer. Perhaps the most likely response involves an interaction between the two factors of individual differences and crowd characteristics. Much research has been completed attempting to answer the primary question posed above, and most of this research has surrounded the theory of social facilitation.

Early research in the area of performance effects due to co-actors or an audience showed contradictory findings. As Dorrance (1973) notes, some studies (Meumann, 1904; Tripplett, 1897) indicated that an audience improved or facilitated performance, while others (Burri, 1931; Ekdahl, 1929; Moore, 1917) noted performance decrements in the presence of others. It was in 1924 that the term *social facilitation* was coined by Gordon Allport. Perhaps due to the contradictory findings and, as Zajonc (1965) suggests, the outbreak of World War II, research in this area severely declined in the late 1930s. It was not until 1965 that Zajonc rekindled the interest in this subject with his influential paper.

In this article, Zajonc (1965) reviews the research to that date, clarifies the concept of social facilitation, and more importantly, offers an explanation as to why the phenomenon occurs. Early in his piece, Zajonc divides social facilitation into two distinct paradigms: audience effects and co-action effects. The first paradigm involves the observation of behavior when it occurs in the presence of passive spectators. The second examines behavior when it occurs in the presence of other individuals engaged in the same activity. Subsequent inquiries have tended to select one of these paradigms, creating essentially two separate tracks of research. Zajonc (1965) continues in his article and develops the drive theory of social facilitation. This explanation was the catalyst to the renewed interest in the field. Just as the two paradigms have created distinct paths of research, so too has the explanatory framework. Perhaps the most prominent explanations are drive theory, Cottrell's (1968) learned drive theory, and the inverted-U theory.

In her thorough report, Dorrance (1973) briefly summarizes the majority of "explanations for underlying causes of social facilitation" (p. 9). These causes include mechanical and physiological reasons, distraction, social reinforcement and punishment, motivation, competition, and arousal. Of these, several review articles (Guerin and Innes, 1982, 1984; Landers and McCullagh, 1976) have indicated that arousal and the subsequent effects on attention are the dominant underlying mechanism on which the larger theories are based. For example, Zajonc's (1965) original application of the Hull-Spence drive theory states that as drive increases, so too does the elicitation of the dominant response to a given task. In the early learning stage of a task, the dominant response is composed of many incorrect decisions. However, as one progresses and becomes an expert at the task, the dominant response is categorized by correct responses and choices. As Zajonc (1965) posits, the influence of an audience or co-actor(s) may serve to increase an individual's arousal level (drive), thus eliciting the dominant response. Therefore, for novices the presence of an audience will increase drive and bring forth the dominant response of incorrect choices, thus decreasing performance. However, the presence of an audience for an expert will increase drive and the likelihood of the correct dominant response, thus enhancing performance.

Despite the fact that Zajonc (1965) based his drive theory explanation on "indirect and scanty" (p. 274) evidence, his ideas have permeated and propelled many research efforts. However, Zajonc's original idea has been questioned and other theories and explanations for the social facilitation phenomenon have emerged. Perhaps the most prominent critic of Zajonc's (1965) views is Cottrell (1968) and his learned drive theory. His contention is that the mere presence of another individual may not be enough to increase one's drive. Rather, a condition of evaluation (potential or actual) is required to augment one's arousal level. This evaluative context integrates a learning component such that drive becomes a learned condition based upon the presence of evaluative others.

Another critic of Zajonc's (1965) views is Glaser (1982). Addressing Zajonc's theory he writes:

> This interpretation is challenged on five main grounds: that it fails to explain adequately the early findings in the field; that the most influential subsequent tests of it are unsatisfactory; that a large number of studies which appear to contradict it have gone uncited and unheeded; that Hull-Spence drive theory is problematic per se; and that its application to the core of social psychology is inappropriate and has led to an impoverished conceptualization of the field (p. 265).

This rather scathing criticism is backed up by the suggestion that researchers take a symbolic interactionist approach to the study of social facilitation. As Glaser (1982) notes, this view maintains that the self is made up of the "reflected appraisals" of others. When performing a task before an audience one receives these appraisals. If the appraisals (real or imagined) are incongruent with one's sense of self a heightened situation of threat, and in turn anxiety, arises. Glaser (1982) goes on to state that this anxiety will affect performance "directly through the Yerkes-Dodson inverted-U relationship" and "indirectly through behaviors and cognitive processes" (p. 276). The Yerkes-Dodson inverted-U law essentially states that arousal and anxiety will facilitate performance up to a certain threshold based upon the task and personal characteristics. However, if arousal increases beyond that threshold, performance quickly deteriorates. An earlier study (Dorrance, 1976) lends support to this view. On a ball rolling task, increases in audience size coincided with increases in arousal, and the performance pattern suggested an inverted-U relationship.

From the brief discussion above, one can clearly see that both sides maintain strong convictions in support of their own theories. While this debate has been beneficial to the generation of research, the lack of unity has hampered our understanding of the social facilitation phenomenon. There is a need for a well controlled, un-biased, quantitative review of the literature to elucidate which theories are the most valid and reliable. While traditional narrative reviews are important and insightful, meta-analyses offer empirical evidence and may be less susceptible to bias. Meta-analysis statistically combines the findings of multiple inquiries within a given topic. Critics of this method have often used the "apples and oranges" argument, stating that trying to combine all the findings of a diverse set of studies is like comparing apples and oranges in terms of the differing populations, methods, and overall qualities of the studies. However, a well devised, controlled, and executed meta-analysis can control for these potential limitations, with the result being a strong summary position of where we stand in our understanding of a given phenomenon.

In 1983, Bond and Titus conducted a meta-analysis of social facilitation. Their all-inclusive investigation included 241 studies from 1927-1982, and included any/all pertinent articles. Their three dependent variables included physiological arousal, performance quantity (speed), and performance quality (accuracy). However, they investigated two very different processes, namely both mental and motor tasks. Perhaps the most useful finding is that their results support Zajonc's (1965) position. The researchers write, "Results from this meta-analysis favor Zajonc's mere presence position: Others who lack the potential to evaluate task performance have reliable effects on physiological arousal, performance speed, and performance accuracy" (Bond and Titus, 1983, p. 283). While this report is comprehensive and is the backbone of the present investigation, perhaps more useful results can be obtained by narrowing the criteria. As Guerin and Innes (1984) write, "It is proposed that what is needed is not a new overall theory of social facilitation but a micro-analysis of different contexts and the behavior changes they elicit, to see which of the many processes are present in which situations" (p. 47).

The purpose of this study was to integrate the most recent (1983-2004) social facilitation research. Unlike the Bond and Titus (1983) investigation, this meta--analysis consisted only of articles and publications relating social facilitation to motor performance. By narrowing the review to a specific focus, it was hypothesized that a stronger effect would be present, and the specific social contexts that facilitate or inhibit motor performance would be extracted. Thus, the specific questions to be answered were: What are the specific social conditions and contexts in which motor performance is facilitated? And, what theory best explains what the research shows?

METHOD

Selection and Inclusion of Studies

In order to ensure a comprehensive review and in line with previous meta-analyses, the data were obtained through three sources: computer database searches, manual searches, and journal sources. The computer database searches included Academic Search Premier (EBSCO) (1982 to the present), MEDLINE (1982 to the present), ERIC Psychology and Behavioral Science Collection (1982 to the present), PSYCHarticles (1982 to the present), PSYCHinfo (1982 to the present), and SPORTdiscus (1982 to the present). 1982 was selected as the starting date due to the publication of Bond and Titus' (1983) meta-analysis. Their exhaustive review contained data obtained through similar sources from 1927-1981. Thus, the present study serves to update and summarize the most recent findings. The keywords for the search consisted of: "audience," "social facilitation," "crowd," "spectator(s)," "mere-presence," "co-action," "performance," "motor performance," "motor behavior," "sport performance," "athletic performance," "motor task," and "choking." In addition to Bond and Titus' (1983) paper, other comprehensive narrative reviews on social facilitation have been published. The reference lists from these reviews were manually searched for pertinent articles. Finally, 19 journals with a likelihood of relevant research were searched from 1982 (or when they began publication) to the present. These journals included: *Psychological Bulletin, Perceptual and Motor Skills, Journal of Personality and Social Psychology, Journal of Motor Behavior, International Journal of Sport Psychology, Research Quarterly, Journal of Experimental Social Psychology, Journal of Personality, Journal of Sport Psychology, The Sport Psychologist, Journal of Applied Sport Psychology, Sociology of Sport Journal, International Review of Sport Sociology, Journal of Sport and Exercise Psychology, Journal of Sport Behavior, Journal of Sport and Social Issues, Motor Control, Human Movement Science, and Journal Social Psychology.*

The two primary criteria for selection were that the study incorporates some aspect of the theory of social facilitation (e.g. evaluation, mere presence, or co-action) and examines some form of motor task. The operational definition of "motor task" for the purposes of this paper was any task that requires the participant to respond to a stimulus using a manual component. Verbal responses were not included, nor were key presses in response to a predominately mental or memory task. However, video games, reaction time trials, and gross motor tasks did meet the selection criteria.

Coding the Data

Each study that met the eligibility requirements above was then coded based upon several characteristics and variables. Bond and Titus (1983) elected to code their data on "5 procedural and 13 substantive variables" (p. 269). This project followed a similar guideline, but organized the coding of data into six broad categories, with several variables under each heading. The first category that was recorded was the date of the study. Next, the paradigm that was tested was classified. Bond and Titus (1983) named this the "role" variable, as it describes the actions of the others in the study (e.g., evaluative others, mere-presence, or co-actors). Following this was a category that described the various study designs. Information under this section included variables describing the control condition - whether subjects are truly alone in the room, or if others (including the experimenter) are present, or if it is possible to tell given the information reported. Other information included the number of other people that are in the room during the experiment, the familiarity of both the audience and the task, the visibility of both the subject and the observers, and the observer status (e.g., peer or expert). Under the next category were subject characteristics, which included demographic information such as age, gender, and occupation. After the subject characteristics, the response characteristics were recorded. Items under this category were task complexity, the type of task, and the quality and quantity of the response. The two dependent variables [response quality (accuracy) and response quantity (speed)] fell under this heading. Finally, a category that examines the quality of the study was incorporated. Information pertaining to test-retest reliability, validity, and internal consistency was documented under this label.

Computation of Effect Size

Glass, McGaw, and Smith (1981), Hedges and Olkin (1985), Cohen (1988), Cooper (1989), and Thomas and French (1986) provide the significant studies and literature describing the statistical analyses and terminology for a meta-analysis. This meta-analysis followed the guidelines set forth by these seminal reports. As such, d statistics were computed as follows: $d = ((M_1-M_2) / SD)*(1\ 3/4(Nc+Ne-2)-1)$, where M_1 is the mean of the experimental group, M_2 is the mean of the control group, and SD is either the standard deviation of the control group or the pooled standard deviation, as outlined and suggested by Thomas and French (1986). Their suggestions indicate using the pooled standard deviation when there is no clear difference between the experimental and control groups; otherwise the control group SD is acceptable.

The second factor in the equation is a correction for small sample sizes, where Nc and Ne are the number of participants in the control group and experimental group, respectively. Hedges and Olkin (1985) indicated that effect sizes tend to be positively biased in studies with small sample sizes. This correction, therefore, produces a far less biased and more precise statistic. When means and standard deviations were not reported, transformation calculations (as stated by Cooper, 1989) were performed so that an equivalent d statistic was obtained through whichever significance test (e.g. t or F) the researchers of a given study used. In these instances *Meta Win* statistical software (Rosenberg, Adams, and Gurevitch, 2000) was used to obtain the statistic. Study variances were then calculated following the formula: $V_d = (Nc+Ne/NcNe) + (d^2/2(Nc+Nc))$, where, again Nc and Ne are the number of participants in the control group and experimental group, respectively, and d is the calculated effect size. Effect sizes (ESs) and variances were first calculated for all individual studies. Next, overall effect sizes and variances were obtained by averaging all of the component studies within a given category/variable. All summary statistics were obtained using the *Meta Win* software and a random-effects design (Rosenberg et al., 2000). For a more detailed description of the formulas and steps in this process, readers are encouraged to reference the reports of Thomas and French (1986) or Hedges and Olkin (1985).

It was necessary to stratify studies according to the moderating variables. For example, under the "paradigm" heading, ESs from articles examining mere presence were averaged under one overall ES, while ESs pertaining to co-action were averaged under another overall ES. The moderating variables were then addressed within one of the three paradigms. This stratification and categorization should serve to control many of the potential limitations and criticisms of meta-analysis.

RESULTS

The literature search produced 79 studies relating some aspect of the theory of social facilitation to motor performance. Of these studies, 39 reported appropriate statistics for analysis. Additionally, the search revealed two phenomena related to social facilitation - social loafing and the home advantage/disadvantage. Separate analyses were performed only on the former phenomenon.

Social Facilitation

Mere Presence

The overall social facilitation ES was .05. While this is a very small statistic (no effect), one should keep in mind that it is composed of all paradigms and moderating variables. As stated above, the social facilitation studies were stratified based upon the specific paradigm being tested (i.e., mere presence, evaluation, or co-action). Table 1 presents all of the summary statistics under the mere presence heading. It should be noted (for all tables) that a significant value ($\leq.05$) in the "prob(X^2)" column "indicates that the variance among effects sizes is greater than expected by sampling error" (Rosenberg et al, 2000, p. 23). The authors go on to state that the total heterogeneity (Qtotal) is tested against a X^2 distribution, with the null hypothesis being that all ESs are equal. Thus, non-significant values are desired because it indicates that sampling error accounts for most of the variance under the variable being studied. Under the mere presence paradigm, the overall ES, based upon 11 studies and 24 individual ESs, proved to be a small effect, with a value of .202. This statistic was further examined in regards to the moderating variables.

Table 1. Mere Presence Summary Statistics

	Mean ES	95% CI	Heterogeneity (Qtotal)	df	Prob (X^2)	t-score	df	p value
High Control Validity	**.4158**	**-.48 to 1.31**	**6.4369**	**5**	**.26599**			
Low Control Validity	.1248	-.33 to .58	18.9842	17	.32944	1.41	22	p>.05
Audience # ≤ 10	.3891	-.08 to .86	19.1686	16	.26002			
Audience # 11+	-.1848	-.71 to .34	5.3409	6	.50089	2.26	22	p<.05
Familiar Audience	-0.790	-.61 to .46	5.9257	6	.43156			
Non-familiar Audience	.3400	-.17 to .85	18.4735	16	.29691	1.94	22	p>.05
Familiar Task	.0623	-.43 to .56	16.7502	15	.33402			
Non-familiar Task	.4509	-.25 to 1.15	8.4994	7	.29062	2.08	22	p<.05
Subject Visible	.2206	-.24 to .68	21.1742	18	.27072			
Subject Not Visible	.1354	-.79 to 1.06	3.7384	4	.44256	.45	22	p>.05
Observer Visible	.2133	-.21 to .64	23.4245	20	.26843			
Observer Not Visible	.1366	-1.53 to 1.81	1.8037	2	.40582	.334	22	p>.05
Observer Stat: Peer	-.2086	-.54 to .12	10.9628	12	.53211			
Observer Stat: Expert	.7028	.03 to 1.38	11.9714	10	.28698	4.85	22	p<.05
Sports Task	-.1146	-.41 to .18	11.5883	12	.47928			
Laboratory Task	.6466	-.07 to 1.36	11.8699	10	.29386	4.07	22	p<.05
Overall	.2020	-.17 to .58	26.9636	23	.25752			

Control group validity was the first variable to be studied. Studies were categorized as either "high" or "low" depending upon whether or not the subject was truly alone (pure test of mere presence) in the room or if someone (usually the experimenter) was present during the control condition. The word "valid" was used solely as a description and is not intended to indicate any connotation of statistics or significance. Thus, highly "valid" control conditions are true tests of the mere presence paradigm, while studies with low "validity" in the control conditions are confounded by the presence of at least one person, usually the experimenter. The results showed that studies with the high (truly alone) control condition validity tended to have a larger effect than those studies with the low (experimenter or others present) control condition validity (ES = .42 and ES = .12, respectively).

Audience size was examined next. Since there was a wide range in the number of audience members, a dichotomous grouping was established based upon the characteristics of the sample. Studies with 10 or fewer audience members were lumped into one group, while audiences of 11 or more members were grouped into another cluster based upon a logical break in the sample. Small facilitation effects seemed to occur only in audiences with 10 or fewer individuals (ES = .39).

Audiences of 11 or more were not associated with either performance enhancement or deterioration (ES = -.18).

Another audience variable, audience familiarity, was coded based upon how familiar the subject was with the audience members. The data indicated that familiar audiences had no effect on motor performance (ES = -.08). However, unfamiliar audiences had a small facilitative effect (ES = .34), with the difference in these two effect sizes approaching statistical significance.

Zajonc's (1965) drive theory explanation of social facilitation revolves around experts and novices. The presence of an audience is hypothesized to facilitate expert performance, while hindering novices' performance on motor tasks. This issue was addressed with the task familiarity variable. Subjects were classified as being familiar with a task if they went through a series of learning trials to reach a baseline criterion or it was stated in the text that they were "skilled". If no mention was made, it was assumed that the task was new, and thus unfamiliar. The results do not directly support Zajonc's (1965) explanation. Familiar tasks (experts) were not affected by the presence of an audience (ES = .06), whereas non-familiar tasks (novices) showed small to moderate facilitation effects (ES = .45). This finding will be addressed in the discussion.

The results from both the visibility of the subject and the visibility of the observer variables were similar and unremarkable. When subjects were visible to observers higher effects were found than when they were not visible (ES = .22 and ES = .13, respectively). Likewise, when observers were visible to subjects, higher effects were found than when the observers were not visible (ES = .21 and ES = .13, respectively). However, these differences were not statistically significant.

While the visibility of the observer had little to no effect on performance, the status of that individual(s) did seem to have an impact. Peer observers were shown to have a small debilitative effect (ES = -.20). Conversely, expert observers had a moderate to strong facilitative effect (ES = .70).

Finally, the last variable to be looked at was the type of task. Tasks were divided into either sport/exercise endeavors or laboratory activities. Laboratory tasks (pursuit rotor, computer tracking, etc.) produced moderate facilitative effects (ES=.64), while the sport/exercise (basketball, baseball, running, etc.) tasks were shown to have no effect (ES=-.11).

Discussion

The results from the mere presence paradigm are logical, though not striking. Further discussion of the control condition validity, audience size, subject visibility, and observer visibility variables is not warranted. The non-existent to small effects stand for themselves. However, as was alluded to earlier, some surprising results were found. The fact that no effect was found for familiar audiences may indicate that performing in a comfortable situation (i.e., in front of individuals one knows) is not a sufficient condition to increase drive, and thus produce the social facilitation effect. Additionally, the finding that the ES was negative may further be a sign that familiar audiences distract attention away from the task at hand, thereby decreasing performance.

This idea is supported by the Distraction/Conflict theory, which states that the presence of others attracts the performer's attention, leading to distraction from the task and decreased performance (Jones and Gerard, 1967). Further, Sanders and Baron (1975) suggest that distraction can increase drive through the conflict between attending to the task and attending to the distraction. This notion is strengthened by the fact that the ES was also negative under the peer observer status variable. Conversely, expert observers generated the strongest ES. Perhaps this is due to their status as experts generating a condition of increased drive, and thus facilitating performance. Of course, this reasoning must be considered within the context of skilled and novice performers. The seemingly contradictory finding that peer observation resulted in a decrease in performance (perhaps due to higher distraction) and the finding that familiar tasks were not affected by an audience (perhaps because they could block out the audience) is explained through the different levels in skill of the participants. When examining observer status, task familiarity was not controlled. Thus, in each level of the observer status variable there were both skilled and novice performers. Similarly, when discussing the task familiarity variable, observer status was not controlled. Thus, in each level of task familiarity variable there were both peer and expert observers. Each dyad was tested against its counterpart, so any conclusions or explanations must remain specific to that individual variable.

The data from the mere presence paradigm does not fully support Zajonc's (1965) theory. Non-familiar (novel) tasks generated small to moderate facilitative effects, while the performance on familiar activities was not affected by the presence of an audience. However, there is a potential confound in the way the familiar tasks were coded. It is possible that tasks were not well learned, even after progressing through a series of trials and reaching a baseline criterion. Thus, the "familiar task" group may contain studies in which individuals were classified as skilled, yet were really novices. If this was the case, instead of seeing facilitative effects, the ES would be smaller than expected, as the present data showed. Future studies should attempt to have a clearer delineation of novice and skilled participants. It may even be necessary to stratify various levels of skills, such that high school, college, and professional athletes' reactions to the presence of an audience can be documented and studied.

Evaluation

The evaluation paradigm was coded such that only those studies indicating that participants were explicitly evaluated, graded, or judged were included. This left a total of seven studies and 11 individual ESs. The overall evaluation ES was moderate and negative (ES = -.51). As with the mere-presence paradigm, evaluation studies were, with two exceptions, examined based upon the same moderating variables. Since subjects were evaluated, they had to be visible. Thus, the visibility of the subject variable was excluded because all studies and individual ESs would have been included. The result from this category would be identical to the overall effect. Additionally, only one study used a familiar audience. Due to this fact, the familiar audience variable was also excluded from further analysis. Table 2 displays all of the summary statistics under this heading.

The results from the control condition validity variable were not remarkable. It is important to note that the ES in the high control condition is only based on two individual ESs. With that fact in mind, no effect (ES = -.19) was found in the high validity situation, while a moderate effect (ES = -.60) was discovered in the low validity group. Similarly, the observer visibility variable produced small to moderate effects, close to the overall ES, with a slightly larger decrease in performance in the visible observer group. It appears that being evaluated, either by a visible or non-visible individual, has a similar negative effect on performance.

The number of individuals in the audience was much smaller under this paradigm than in the mere presence group. In fact, only one study investigated the effects of an audience greater than 10. This study was excluded, thus creating only one audience group of ≤10. Not surprisingly, the ES was moderate and negative (ES = -.54). This same study was also the only study to examine the effects of a familiar audience. The small individual ES (-.20) from that study was removed from further analyses, eliminating the familiar audience condition. Thus, the ESs for both the audience number and non-familiar audience variables are the same.

The effect of observer status showed a similar trend as in the mere presence paradigm. Peer observers/evaluators had no effect on subsequent performance (ES= -.04), while expert evaluators caused a moderate to large (ES = -.78) deterioration. Again, peer evaluation may not have created a condition of increased drive, effectively neutralizing the phenomenon.

The two variables that revealed the most interesting findings were the type of task and task familiarity. Because of the small number of studies, the type of task and task familiarity variables overlapped, again giving identical statistics. Laboratory (unfamiliar) type motor tasks produced the largest ES (-.93) of the group. A much smaller ES (-.26) was revealed for the sport (familiar) type tasks. What is interesting about these findings is that the sport studies usually examined members on a collegiate athletic team (who are highly skilled at their task), while laboratory tests were conducted with a more general student population (novices). The pattern of results is similar to what one would expect to find under Cottrell's (1968) theory. The experts' performance was less negatively affected by the audience, while novices' performance suffered greatly.

Discussion

The results from these analyses lend some support to Cottrell's (1968) learned drive theory. Thus far, it appears that the mere presence of an individual does not have as strong an effect as evaluation on motor performance. Unfortunately, these findings are based on a small sample size and must be interpreted in that light. However, the consistency of the findings (all ESs under evaluation were negative) and the pattern of results are encouraging.

Table 2. Evaluation Summary Statistics

	Mean ES	95% CI	Heterogeneity (Qtotal)	df	Prob (X^2)	t-score	df	p value
High Control Validity	-1.879	-4.35 to 3.97	1.00	1	.31731			
Low Control Validity	-.5986	-1.38 to .18	8.2474	8	.40968	1.56	9	p>.05
Audience # $\leq$ 10	-.5416	-1.22 to .13	10.0904	9	.34322			
Non-familiar Audience	-.5416	-1.22 to .13	10.0904	9	.34322			
Familiar Task	-.2639	-.61 to .08	3.5639	6	.73545			
Non-familiar Task	-.9370	-3.11 to 1.24	3.9094	3	.27142	3.11	9	p<.05
Observer Visible	-.5397	-1.55 to .47	7.4788	6	.27882			
Observer Not Visible	-.4541	-1.07 to .16	.7038	3	.87230	.369	9	p>.05
Observer Stat: Peer	-0.459	-.86 to .76	2.9569	3	.39832			
Observer Stat: Expert	-.7820	-1.72 to .15	6.7842	6	.34127	3.28	9	p<.05
Sports Task	-.2639	-.61 to .08	3.5639	6	.73545			
Laboratory Task	-.9370	-3.11 to 1.24	3.9094	3	.27142	3.11	9	p<.05
Overall	-.5091	-1.11 to .09	11.3637	10	.32989			

Table 3. Co-action Summary Statistics

	Mean ES	95% CI	Heterogeneity (Qtotal)	df	Prob (X²)	t-score	df	p value
High Control Validity	.6364	-.01 to 1.28	2.879	3	.4076			
Low Control Validity	.0435	-2.88 to 2.86	1	1	.31731	2.13	4	p>.05
Subject & Observer Visible	.2575	-1.4 to .66	3.0152	3	.38929			
Subject & Observer Not Visible	1.1236	-2.83 to 5.08	.0581	1	.80946	2.53	4	p>.05
Simple Task	.1285	-4.63 to 4.89	1	1	.31731			
ComplexTask	.5575	-.11 to 1.22	3.5180	3	.31843	1.45	4	p<.05
Overall	.4267	-.025 to .88	6.1517	5	.29174			

Co-Action

Co-action was the final paradigm under the social facilitation heading to be considered and was defined as two individuals working simultaneously on the same task. The overall co-action ES (.43) was in the small to moderate range and was based on four studies and six individual ESs. Table 3 presents the co-action summary statistics. Due to the small number of available ESs and similarities between studies, many of the moderating variables could not be addressed.

The control group validity variable once again showed that the high validity control condition tended to be associated with larger effects than the low validity group (ES =.63 and ES = .04, respectively). Similar disparities in the differences of ESs between dyads were found for all tested variables. Both visible subjects and visible observers shared the same individual ESs, as did the non-visible subject and non-visible observer variables. Thus, the two variables were combined under one visible vs. non-visible dyad. The visibility effect was only slightly facilitative (ES= .26), whereas the non-visibility effect was highly facilitative (ES=1.1) . Also noteworthy is the difference in task complexity. Working on a complex task with a co-actor (ES= .55) tends to increase performance over working with a co-actor on a simple task (ES= .13), which seems to have no effect.

Discussion

The large differences between the visible and non-visible conditions may be indicative of a fear of performing worse than the co-actor. When performing in the presence of co-actor, one can gauge individual performance simply by monitoring the other performer. However, when performance norms are unavailable (non-visible condition), and one cannot tell if he/she is performing up to par, the fear of being labeled "below average" may be enough to increase drive and facilitate, or hinder, subsequent performance. As for task complexity, simple tasks may not hold performers' attention as well as complex tasks do; nor may they elicit the same desire for social comparison as complex tasks. The need for social comparison, therefore, may be the stimulus for increasing drive and performance outcomes. This paradigm leads directly into the related field of social loafing.

Social Loafing

Five studies, yielding 17 ESs, were included in the social loafing analysis. Social loafing (also known as the Ringelmann Effect as cited by Latane, Williams and Harkins, 1979) is defined as the tendency for individual performance to decrease in a group, such that group performance is substantially less than the sum of individual performances. Individual ESs were calculated using group performance as the experimental mean and individual performance as the control mean. By setting up the formula in this way, if individual performance exceeded group performance, a negative value would result. Thus, any negative ES is indicative of the social loafing phenomenon. Similarly, a more negative value is representative of a larger effect.

The results confirmed that social loafing seems to exist. The overall mean ES of -.26 falls into the "small" range of Cohen's (1988) classification. This effect appears to be fairly constant between males and females. When controlling for gender, the resulting ESs were -.26 for males and -.19 for females.

Discussion

Even though the resulting ESs represent small effects, it is again encouraging that the results are consistent. One would not expect to find large differences between males and females, nor should those values be different from the overall effect. It is important to keep in mind that these statistics are based upon five studies and 17 individual ESs. With these low numbers one must be cautious when drawing any meaningful conclusions. Future studies should address this issue. It seems reasonable to conclude, however, that individual performance often exceeds that of performance within a group.

GENERAL DISCUSSION

The purpose of this study was to review the most recent social facilitation literature and identify the specific social contexts which bolster or hinder motor performance. Another goal was to evaluate which theory best explains the trends found in the data. The results from the mere-presence paradigm generally revealed small to moderate effects indicating the presence of an individual does facilitate performance, but only slightly (ES=.20). One of the most striking findings occurred under the task familiarity variable in which novice performers (non-familiar task) experienced facilitation effects in the presence of an audience, while skilled performers (familiar task) did not receive any benefit. Another noteworthy result indicated that peer observers had small debilitative effects on performance, whereas expert observers elicited moderate to large facilitation.

The evaluation paradigm also showed moderate effects. Interestingly, all effect sizes were negative, meaning that the presence of an evaluative other decreased performance across all conditions. For the purpose of this study, the most telling statistics were found under the task familiarity, observer status, and task type variables. When the task was familiar (skilled performers) evaluative audiences only had a small debilitative effect on performance. However, non-familiar (novel) tasks performed under evaluation showed large performance decreases. Apparently, familiarity with a task mitigated the negative effects of evaluation. A similar pattern emerged under the observer status variable. Expert evaluators were associated with moderate to large performance declines, while peer evaluators had no effect on performance. Evaluation by an expert tended to negatively impact performance, while peer evaluation, perhaps perceived as less threatening, had no negative impact. Finally, performance on sport tasks was only slightly hampered, yet performance on laboratory motor tasks suffered large negative effects during evaluation. Perhaps the familiarity of sports tasks made evaluation less negatively charged, while laboratory motor tasks, by definition not in a particularly familiar setting, elicited large negative effects on performance.

Another paradigm, the co-action paradigm, was limited by a small sample size, and thus the worth of the results is questionable. An extension of this paradigm is the social loafing literature, which showed an interesting facilitating effect. As with the mere presence paradigm, small to moderate facilitation effects occurred when working with another individual on the same task. While facilitation effects were found for one co-actor, groups of co-actors lead to social loafing. There was a small overall social loafing effect that was fairly constant between males and females.

Returning to the goals of this report, the main finding that evaluation caused a decline in motor performance lends some support to Cottrell's (1968) learned drive theory. Recall that his theory states that evaluation is necessary to increase arousal level, thus making drive a learned response. Experts experienced a decline in performance (contrary to theory predictions), but this decline was marked by a small effect size (-.26). Alternatively (and in accordance with Cottrell's statements), non-skilled individuals suffered large (ES = -.94) performance declines when being evaluated. While social facilitation was not demonstrated, the fact that the experts did not experience the same severity of performance decline as did the novices is in the predicted direction. Essentially, the presence of an evaluative audience resulted in drastic performance deterioration for novices, but only small declines for experts. Further, these evaluation effects were much stronger when the evaluator was an expert, as opposed to a peer.

As previously stated, Zajonc's (1965) drive theory was not substantiated. The mere presence of another individual did facilitate novice performance, but had no effect on expert performance. This finding is the opposite of what Zajonc's (1965) theory would have predicted. As noted above, increased drive should result in the elicitation of the dominant response. For novices this response consists of incorrect movements. Thus, in the presence of an audience, drive increases, incorrect decisions and movements are evoked, and performance decreases. It is possible, as mentioned earlier that audiences made up of peer observers are not a condition that increases one's drive. If drive is not increased, the incorrect dominant response would not be elicited, and performance would be largely unaffected.

Taken together, the results from this analysis provide new insight into the social facilitation effect. Although this analysis was similar to Bond and Titus' (1983) paper, it is difficult to draw direct comparisons because different aspects of the social facilitation phenomenon were assessed. However, some similarities do exist. For example, in both studies the magnitudes of effect sizes were generally in the small to moderate range of Cohen's (1988) classification. Additionally, several variables showed a similar pattern of results. The control condition "validity" variable in both studies tended to report larger effect sizes when the subject was truly alone (high validity). This finding is logical in that better controlled and more thoughtfully planned studies often show greater effects. Another variable that was found to corroborate Bond and Titus' (1983) report was the observer status category. They write, "...familiar others have smaller effects than unfamiliar others in all six of the comparisons..." (p. 280). As affirmed earlier, comparable results were also found in this study. The idea that peer observers may not increase drive is based upon the distraction/conflict theory (Jones and Gerard, 1967).

Although such variables as observer and subject visibility and the number of audience members are interesting and provide unique insight into the various social conditions that facilitate or hinder motor performance, the crux of the matter lies within the various paradigms, task familiarity, and type of task variables. Differences emerged between this study and Bond and Titus' (1983) conclusions in regards to these variables. As stated in the introduction, the researchers found support for Zajonc's (1965) drive theory. In the present endeavor, Cottrell's (1968) learned drive theory seems to better explain the results. In the evaluative context, much more robust effect sizes, in line with his theory, were found. This finding was strengthened through the type of task variable that showed sports tasks, consisting primarily of skilled participants, had less performance decreases than individuals completing novel tasks. It was not unexpected that this difference would occur. The Bond and Titus (1983) investigation primarily consisted of cognitive activities whereas this review concentrated exclusively on motor tasks. Because mental and motor responses are two separate (but related) channels, it is reasonable to assume that the overt action associated with a motor response is susceptible to different (but related) stressors than the intrinsic processes of a mental task. This could explain why the Bond and Titus (1983) investigation resulted in Zajonc's (1965) explanation being favored, whereas this study supports Cottrell's (1968) theory.

There is also another explanation that better describes the results reported here that has largely gone either unnoticed or unheeded in the literature. Sanders (1981) proposed the Attentional Processes model in which the three leading theories (mere presence drive theory, learned drive theory, and distraction/conflict) are slightly modified and combined. Sanders' (1981) contention is that the mere presence and learned drive theory explanations are "antecedents leading to the attentional conflict described by the D/C explanation" (p. 245). He proposes that the mere presence assumption be modified from a "drive-inducing alertness reflex" to a "drive-neutral orienting reflex" (p.245). Thus, the presence of an audience may be significant, but does not necessarily increase drive. Rather, the orienting reflex serves as a monitoring system to either keep attending to the audience or to the task. He suggests a similar modification to the learned drive theory, where the "drive-inducing anticipation of rewards and punishments" is changed to "a drive-neutral learned motivation for attending to others" (p. 246). Again, this would have the effect of acting as a monitoring system. If information can be gleaned from the audience, attention and drive are increased to those individuals. Conversely, if no information can be acquired, attention is directed at the task and no increase in drive occurs.

The results from this study generally lend support to this model. In the mere presence paradigm peer observation resulted in a decline in performance, while observation by experts facilitated performance. Under the Attentional Processes model, it can be said that peer observers captured more attention from the participants than did the expert observers. Experts may have been viewed as individuals who will never been seen again, whereas peers are friends and people who may be seen on a regular basis, and thus social comparisons and competition may influence the amount of devoted attention. Further support comes from the evaluation paradigm, although the results are the inverse of the mere presence data. Again, the apparent conflict between the mere presence and evaluation paradigms can be conceptualized if one maintains that the two groups (mere presence and evaluation) are distinct. Overt evaluation is a different situation than inferred evaluation. In inferred evaluation, peer observation may attract more of the participant's attention because no concrete statements about performance quality are proffered. Thus, performance norms only reside in the participant's thinking and social comparisons. However, when overt performance feedback is being offered, it is logical that experts would carry more weight than a peer. As such, in this paradigm, peer evaluation may not be as attentionally consuming as expert evaluation. Peer evaluation may have less meaning for the individual than the feedback from an expert. Again, the pattern of results is consistent with this line of reasoning. Peer evaluators had no effect on performance, indicating attention was devoted to the task, while expert evaluation resulted in a large performance decline, suggesting attention was given to the evaluator.

More support for the model comes from the task familiarity variable. Zajonc's (1965) theory expects experts to perform better in the presence of an audience. The Attentional Processes model does not directly address this issue. However, skilled performers, by definition, would not devote attention to the audience; they would have learned to focus on the task at hand and block out all other distractions. In fact, Williams and Krane (1998) list "a narrow focus of attention concentrated on the activity itself" as a characteristic of the ideal performance state that often leads to peak performance. Therefore, one can assume that neither facilitation effects nor performance decreases would be present. Essentially, there would be no effect. The results from this meta analysis support this view. For both the mere presence and evaluation paradigms, no effect was found for expert performance.

A potential drawback of the model is that it does not address the facilitation effects found for novice performers. If attention was devoted to the audience, as the model would predict, attentional conflict would lead to increased drive, the elicitation of the dominant response, and decreased performance. The results from this study do not support such a scenario. Novice performance was facilitated in the presence of an audience. It is possible that other variables such as motivation, competition and personality characteristics are responsible for this finding.

Taken together, the results from this study suggest that overt expert evaluation causes performance decreases in both skilled and novice performers, and that this effect is more pronounced for the novices. Despite the reported limitations of the Attentional Processes model, it still remains as a viable explanation of the research findings and serves to integrate and unite the social facilitation literature into one track. Clearly, the factors that govern successful performance are numerous and interact complexly. The findings of this study suggest that the role of evaluation in performance is a critical one that needs more examination so that both novices and experts can benefit from the process of being evaluated. The examination of the specific social contexts that facilitate or hamper motor performance should be further explored so that the understanding can be applied to enhance performance at all levels of expertise.

There is a cliché that states, "Nothing succeeds like success." This study suggests the truth of that axiom. Expert performers who have successfully attained a high level of performing are not as negatively affected by audiences or evaluators and can maintain motivation and focus during motor performance. On the other hand, novice participants are more vulnerable to negative effects from evaluation, may not be as able to capitalize on the home advantage, and may be more likely to choke. Their motivation is also more likely to be negatively impacted from competition. This study suggests that one of the challenges of sport psychology is to find ways to help novices reach a level of proficiency that will enable them to feel and become successful, and thus enable them to tap into the synergy that success creates. Research then would find applications that could enrich lives and improve our understanding of the complex interactions of phenomena such as social facilitation, motivation, competition, home advantage, choking, and evaluation.

No study is perfect, and the present report is no exception. Due to the necessity of stratifying studies across the numerous moderating variables, many of the effect sizes were based on small sample sizes. Unfortunately there was no way to control for this, and thus the results must be viewed cautiously. A larger sample size would lend more confidence to the findings and allow for a more reliable understanding of the phenomenon. However, the consistency of the results and the fact that the pattern is in accordance with a prevailing theory may help alleviate concerns.

Another limitation lies in the fact that this report only consisted of published studies, and is thus vulnerable to the "file drawer problem." Glass, McGraw and Smith (1981) write, "....findings reported in journals are, on the average, one-third standard deviation more disposed toward the favored hypothesis of the investigators than findings reported in theses or dissertations" (p. 67). Therefore, it is possible that the ESs are artificially inflated, but the fact that the numbers are comparable to the Bond and Titus (1983) paper, which included both published and unpublished studies, may indicate that any publication bias that exists is minimal.

Despite these limitations, the strength of this analysis lies in its narrow focus and comparable results. Although *small* sample size *and* publication bias may limit the usefulness of the findings, it is important to remember that similar magnitudes of effects were obtained through Bond and Titus' (1983) work. Additionally, by focusing solely on motor tasks, the specific social contexts which affect motor behavior were described. Another strength of this study is that it identified, although by accident, flaws in the reporting of findings.

The goal and importance of this research was to provide a context in which future research can proceed and advance. During the coding process, it became abundantly clear that many studies are not carefully constructed. Often figures presented in tables contradict what was written in the text, or essential statistics were not reported. This led to a lot of expended time and effort searching for and calculating the necessary results. Higher and more consistent standards would facilitate advancements, thus consolidating present understanding and suggesting new directions for research. Meta-analysis can offer a convenient way to summarize the current understanding of a particular topic. However, the results of any analysis are only as good as the component studies. There is a positive trend that several journals now require the inclusion of estimates of effect size with the findings, and this should continue.

REFERENCES[*]

*Anshel M.H. (1995). Examining social loafing among elite female rowers as a function of task duration and mood. *Journal of Sport Behavior, 18(1)*, 39-50.

*Bell, P.A., Loomis, R.J., and Cervone, J.C. (1982). Effects of heat, social facilitation, sex differences, and task difficulty on reaction time. *Human Factors, 24(1)*, 19-24.

Bond, C.F. and Titus, L.J. (1983). Social Facilitation: A meta-analysis of 241 studies. *Psychological Bulletin, 94(2)*, 265-292.

*Bray, S.R. (1999). The home advantage from an individual team perspective. *Journal of Applied Sport Psychology, 11*, 116-125.

*Bray, S.R., Law, J., and Foyle, J. (2003). Team quality and game location effects in English professional soccer. *Journal of Sport Behavior, 26(4)*, 319-334.

Burri, C. (1931). The influences of an audience upon recall. *Journal of Educational Psychology, 22*, 683-690.

*Butler, J.L. and Baumeister, R.F. (1998). The trouble with friendly faces: Skilled performance with a supportive audience. *Journal of Personality and Social Psychology, 75(5)*, 1213-1230.

Cohen, J. (1988). *Statistical power analysis for the behavioral sciences* (2nd ed.). New Jersey: Lawrence Erlbaum.

Cooper, H.M. (1989). *Integrating Research: A Guide for Literature Reviews* (2nd ed.). London, UK: Sage.

---

[*] References marked with an asterisk indicate studies included in the meta-analysis.

*Corston, R. and Colman, A.M. (1996). Gender and social facilitation effects on computer competence and attitudes toward computers. *Journal of Educational Computing Research, 14(2),* 171-183.

Cotttrell, N.B., Sekerak, G.J., Rittle, R.H., and Eack, D.L. (1968). Social facilitatation of dominant responses by the presence of an audience and the mere presence of others. *Journal of Personality and Social Psychology,* 9, 245-250.

*Dandy, J., Brewer, N., and Tottman, R. (2001). Self-consciousness and performance decrements within a sporting context. *The Journal of Social Psychology, 141(1),* 150-152.

Dorrance, P.D. (1973). *Social facilitation and motor performance: Drive summation or inverted-U?* Unpublished master's thesis, University of Washington, Seattle.

*Dube, S.K. and Tatz, S.J. (1991). Audience effects in tennis performance. *Perceptual and Motor Skills, 73,* 844-846.

*Duffy, L.J., and Hinwood, D.P. (1997). Home field advantage: Does anxiety contribute? *Perceptual and Motor Skills, 84,* 283-286.

Ekdahl, A.G. (1929). Effects of attitude on free word association time. *Genetic Psychology Monograph, 5,* 253-338.

*Everett, J.J, Smith, R.E., and Williams, K.D. (1992). Effects of team cohesion and identifiablility on social loafing in relay swimming performance. *International Journal of Sport Psychology, 23,* 311-324.

*Gayton, W.F. and Langevin, G. (1992). Home advantage: Does it exist in individual sports. *Perceptual and Motor Skills, 74,* 706.

*Geisler, G. and Leith, L.M. (1997). The effects of self esteem, self-efficacy, and audience presence on soccer penalty shot performance. *Journal of Sport Behavior, 20(3),* 322-338.

Glaser, A.N. (1982). Drive theory of social facilitation: A critical reappraisal. *British Journal of Social Psychology, 21(4),* 265-282.

Glass, G.V., McGaw, B., and Smith, M.L. (1981). *Meta-analysis in Social Research.* Beverly Hills, CA: Sage.

*Graydon, J. and Murphy, T. (1995). The effect of personality on social facilitation whilst performing a sports related task. *Personality and Individual Differences, 19(2),* 265-267.

*Guerin, B. (1988). Reducing evaluation effects in mere presence. *The Journal of Social Psychology, 129(2),* 183-190.

Guerin, B., and Innes, J.M. (1982). Social facilitation and social monitoring: A new look at Zajonc's mere presence hypothesis. *British Journal of Social Psychology, 21,* 7-18.

Guerin, B., and Innes, J.M. (1984). Explanations of social facilitation: A review. *Current Psychological Research and Reviews, 3(2), 32-52.*

Hedges, L.V. and Olkin, I. (1985). *Statistical methods for meta-analysis.* New York, NY: Academic Press.

*Hollifield, N.L. (1982). Effect of prior performance experience before audiences on a dominant and nondominant motor response. *Journal of Sport Psychology, 4,* 317-323.

*Huddleston, S., Doody, S.G., and Ruder, M.K. (1985). The effect of prior knowledge of the social loafing phenomenon on performance in a group. *International Journal of Sport Psychology, 16,* 176-182.

Jones, E. and Gerard, H. (1967). *Foundations of social psychology.* New York, NY: Wiley.

*Kimble, C.E. and Rezabek, J.S. (1992). Playing games before an audience: Social facilitation or choking. *Social Behavior and Personality, 20(2),* 115-120.

Latane, B., Williams, K.D., and Harkins, S.G. (1979). Many hands make light work: The causes and consequences of social loafing. *Journal of Personality and Social Psychology, 37,* 823-832.

*Law, J., Masters, R., Bray, S.R., Eves, F, and Bardswell, I. (2003). Motor performance as a function of audience affability and metaknowledge. *Journal of Sport and Exercise Psychology, 25,* 484-500.

Landers, D.M. and McCullagh, P. (1976). Social facilitation of motor performance. *Exercise Sport Science Review, 4,* 125-162.

*McCutcheon, L.E. (1984). The home advantage in high school athletics. *Journal of Sport Behavior, 7(4),* 135-138.

*Miller, Q.L. (1989). The effects of social facilitation on persons performing a manual work task. *Occupational Therapy in Mental Health, 9(3),* 2 1-30.

Meumann, E. (1904). Haus and Schularbeit: Experimente an kinder der volkschule. *Die Deutsche Schule, 8,* 279-303, 337-359, 416-431. Cited by Zajonc, R.B. (1966) *Social psychology: An experimental approach.* Belmont, CA: Brooks/Cole Publishing Co.

Moore, H.T. (1917). Laboratory tests of anger, fear, and sex interests. *American Journal of Psychology, 8,* 131-134.

*Moore, J.C. and Brylinsky, J.A. (1993). Spectator effect on team performance in college basketball. *Journal of Sport Behavior, 16(2),* 77-85.

*Moore, J.C. and Brylinsky, J. (1995). Facility familiarity and the home advantage. *Journal of Sport Behavior, 18(4),* 302-312.

*Murray, J.F. (1983). Effects of alone and audience on motor performance for males and females. *International Journal of Sport Psychology*, 14, 92-97.

*Piche, A. and Sachs, M. (1982). Influence of friendship on performance on a noncompetitive task. *Perceptual and Motor Skills, 54,* 1212-1214.

*Pickens, M. (1994). Game location as a determinant of team performance in acc basketball during 1900-1991. *Journal of Sport Behavior, 17(4),* 212-217.

*Rhea, M.R., Landers, D.M., Alvar, B.A., and Arent, S.M. (2003). The effects of competition and the presence of an audience on weight lifting performance. *Journal of Strength and Conditioning Research, 17(2),* 303-306.

Rosenberg, M.S., Adams, D.C., Gurevitch, J. (2000). *Meta Win: Statistical software for meta-analysis, version 2.* Sunderland, MA: Sinauer Associates.

*Salminen S. (1993). The effect of the audience on the home advantage. *Perceptual and Motor Skills, 76,* 1123-1128.

Sanders, G.S. (1981). Driven by distraction: An integrative review of social facilitation theory and research. *Journal of Experimental Social Psychology, 17,* 227-251.

Sanders, G.S. and Baron, R.S. *(1975).* The motivating effects of distraction on task performance. *Journal of Personality and Social Psychology, 32,* 956-963.

*Sawyer, D.T. and Noel, F.J. (2000). Effect of an audience on learning a novel motor skill. *Perceptual and Motor Skills, 91,* 539-545.

Silva III, J.M. and Andrew, J.A. (1987). An analysis of game location and basketball performance in the atlantic coast conference. *International Journal of Sport Psychology, 18,* 188-204.

*Smith, D.R. (2003). The home advantage revisited. *Journal of Sport and Social Issues,* 27(4), 346-371.

*Swain, A. (1996). Social loafing and Identifiably: The mediating role of achievement goal orientations. *Research Quarterly for Exercise and Sport, 67(3),* 337-344.

*Terry, D.J. and Kearnes, M. (1993). Effects of an audience on the task performance of subjects with high and low self-esteem. *Personality and Individual Differences, 15(2),* 137-145.

Thomas, J.R., and French, K.E. (1986). The use of meta-analysis in exercise and sport: A tutorial. *Research Quarterly for Exercise and Sport, 57(3),* 196-204.

Tripplett, N. (1897). The dynamogenic factors in pace-keeping and competition. *American Journal of Psychology, 9, 507-533.*

*Watson II, J.C. and Krantz III, A.J. (2003). Home field advantage: New stadium construction and team performance in professional sports. *Perceptual and Motor Skills, 97,* 794-796.

*Weinstein I., Prather, G.A., and De Man, A.F. (1987). College baseball pitchers' throwing velocities as a function of awareness of being clocked. *Perceptual and Motor skills, 64,* 1185-1186.

*White S.A. (1991). Effects of gender and competitive coaction on motor performance. *Perceptual and Motor Skills, 73,* 581-582.

Williams, J.M. and Krane, V. (1998). Psychological characteristics of peak performance. In J.M. Williams (Ed.), *Applied sport psychology* (pp. 158-170). Mountain View, CA: Mayfield.

*Worringham, C.J. and Messick, D.M. (1983). Social facilitation of running: An unobtrusive study. *The Journal of Social Psychology, 121,* 23-29.

*Wright, E.F. (1991). The home-course disadvantage in golf championships: Further evidence for the undermining effect of supportive audiences on performance under pressure. *Journal of Sport Behavior, 14(1),* 51-61.

Zajonc, R.B. *(1965).* Social facilitation. *Science, 149,* 269-274.

In: Sports and Athletics Developments
Editor: James H. Humphrey, pp. 29-44

ISBN: 978-1-60456-205-7
© 2008 Nova Science Publishers, Inc.

Chapter 2

USE OF PROACTIVE PESSIMISM AS A COPING STRATEGY FOR SPORT FANS: THE IMPORTANCE OF TEAM IDENTIFICATION

Daniel L. Wann[*] *and Frederick G. Grieve*[**]
[*]Murray State University
[**]Western Kentucky University

ABSTRACT

We examined use of proactive (i.e., defensive) pessimism as a strategy employed by sport fans to assist them in coping with the possibility that their team will perform poorly. Proactive pessimism occurs as persons become more pessimistic about a self-relevant event as the event draws near. This suggests that fans may become more pessimistic about their team's chances of success as a season approaches. Use of this strategy was expected to be most prominent among fans with a high level of team identification for whom use of the strategy would be beneficial. However, these fans were not expected to lower their feelings of connection to the team as the season approached. Finally, we examined the potential impact of proactive pessimism on behavioral intentions (i.e., desire to attend the team's games). Participants completed a questionnaire packet four weeks prior to the start of the Major League Baseball season and then again one week prior. The packet assessed demographics, level of identification with one's favorite baseball team, and expectations for and excitement about the upcoming season. The results confirmed the expected pattern of effects as highly identified fans (but not those low in identification) reported lowered expectations at Time 2 relative to Time 1 (i.e., they became proactively pessimistic). Also as expected, there was no Time 1 to Time 2 change in connections to the team. Finally, the results indicated that lowly identified fans expressed greater interest in attending the team's games as the season approached while highly identified fans exhibited the opposite pattern.

For a number of decades, social scientific researchers have documented the psychological well-being benefits of group membership (e.g., Cohen and Wills, 1985; Hogg and Abrams, 1990; Linville, 1987; Rowe and Kahn, 1998). For instance, the social support provided by group membership has been found to aid in the psychological health of individuals in stigmatized groups (Crocker and Major, 1989), religious organizations (Diener and Clifton, 2002), school peer groups (Brown and Lohr, 1987), and members of the deaf community (Bat-Chava, 1993, 1994), to name but a few. In fact, the benefits of group membership are so robust that, based on his review of this literature, Compton (2005, p. 48) concluded that "positive social relationships" were one of the "core variables that best predict happiness and satisfaction with life" (i.e., psychological well-being).

Within the last two decades, a number of sport scientists have argued that one should be able to replicate the aforementioned pattern of effects among sport fans. Theoretically, the social nature of this activity should result in well-being benefits among fans (Melnick, 1993; Smith, 1988; Wann, Melnick, Russell, and Pease, 2001; Zillmann, Bryant, and Sapolsky, 1989). However, according to the Team Identification – Social Psychological Health Model (Wann, in press), the key to acquiring well-being benefits via sport fandom is not a function of mere sport fandom (i.e., simply possessing an interest in a player, team, or sport). Rather, according to this framework, fans will exhibit improved social psychological health when they possess high levels of identification with a team (i.e., a strong psychological connection to the team, see Wann et al., 2001), and the identification results in greater social connections to others. These increased social connections are then thought to result in more positive levels of well-being. Empirical evidence for Wann's model is strong. Research indicates that high levels of team identification with teams with readily available social connections are positively associated with many indices of social psychological well-being including loneliness, alienation, collective self-esteem, and social life satisfaction (Wann, Dimmock, and Grove, 2003; Wann, Inman, Ensor, Gates, and Caldwell, 1999; Wann and Pierce, 2005; see Wann, in press, for a complete review of this literature).

Although Wann's (in press) model examines the positive social psychological benefits stemming from team identification, his framework also includes the impact of identity threat and the corresponding attempts to cope with the threat. That is, although the aforementioned literature supports the positive relationship between identification and well-being, it is quite evident both anecdotally and through empirical research (Schwarz, Strack, Kommer, and Wagner, 1987; Wann, Dolan, McGeorge, and Allison, 1994; Wann, Friedman, McHale, and Jaffe, 2003; Wann, Schrader, and Adamson, 1998) that fans often experience negative affect and depression subsequent to watching their team perform poorly. The team's substandard play serves as a threat to the social identity of those fans with a strong allegiance to the team. According to Wann's model, fans have developed numerous methods of coping with the threat of poor team performance which allow them to return to a positive state of well-being. Recent research has documented a number of these strategies including biased attributions (Wann and Dolan, 1994a; Wann and Schrader, 2000; Wann and Wilson, 2001), biased predictions of future and recollections of past team performance (Dietz-Uhler and Murrell, 1999; Markman and Hirt, 2002; Wann and Dolan, 1994b), and biased evaluations of fellow and rival fans (Wann and Branscombe, 1995; Wann and Dolan, 1994c; Wann and Grieve, 2005).

It should be noted that use of these strategies is only found among persons with high levels of team identification. For fans with low levels of identification, unsuccessful team performance is not perceived as a threat because the role of team follower is only a peripheral component of their social identity (Branscombe, Ellemers, Spears, and Doosje, 1999; Wann, in press). As a result, people with low identification are unlikely to report negative affective reactions to poor team performance (i.e., feel threatened) and, hence, do not require the use of coping strategies (Hirt, Zillmann, Erickson, and Kennedy, 1992). Rather, it is the combination of identity threat and high levels of group identification that prompt the use of coping mechanisms (see Ouwerkerk, Ellemers, and de Gilder, 1999; Spears, Doosje, and Ellemers, 1997).

An additional method of coping utilized by sport fans involves the adoption of a pessimistic perception of the team. One form of pessimism, referred to as retroactive pessimism, occurs when fans, subsequent to watching their team fail, adopt the belief that their team never really had a chance from the start. By retrospectively becoming pessimistic about their team's initial chances, fans are better able to cope with the team's loss. Tykocinski, Pick, and Kedmi (2002) provided support for this coping strategy among soccer fans. These researchers found that fans of a defeated team lowered their post-game estimates of success relative to their pre-game estimates. No such shifts were reported by fans of the winning team (they had no need to cope because they were not threatened). Wann, Grieve, and Martin (2006) replicated Tykocinski et al.'s work among basketball fans and found that use of retroactive pessimism was only prominent among highly identified fans.

A second form of pessimism, termed proactive (or defensive) pessimism, is the focus of the current investigation. According to Sheppard, Ouellette, and Fernandez (1996), proactive pessimism occurs as people become more pessimistic about a self-relevant event as the event draws near. These authors documented proactive pessimism among college students; the students lowered estimates of their performance on an exam as the test date approached. Although proactive pessimism had yet to be empirically applied to sport fans, the results provided by Sheppard and his colleagues suggest that fans should become more pessimistic about their team's chances of success as a season approaches. However, as with retroactive pessimism (Wann et al., 2006) and the other coping strategies mentioned above, one would not expect all fans to exhibit significant levels of proactive pessimism. Rather, this strategy should be most apparent among fans with a high level of team identification for whom use of the strategy would be beneficial. Therefore, it was hypothesized (Hypothesis 1) that sport fans would lower their evaluations of their team's chances for a successful season as the season approached and that this pattern of effects would be most prominent among highly identified fans (i.e., a level of identification by time two-way interaction was predicted).

Although changes in evaluations and expectations were predicted, we did not expect the participants to report significant changes in the extent to which they felt psychologically connected to the team. Numerous studies have found that interest in and connection to a team (typically operationalized as team identification) is extremely stable and is rarely impacted by game outcome (Wann, 1996, 2000; Wann et al., 1994). Thus, we did not expect the same changes for interest that we predicted for evaluations. Rather, we hypothesized (Hypothesis 2) that there would *not* be a significant change in psychological connection as a season approached. Psychological connection to the team was assessed in two ways: via team identification and via the extent to which each participant believed that the team in question was his or her favorite team. By combining Hypotheses 1 and 2, we are expecting that fans will proactively cope with the threat of a potentially poor season by lowering their expectations for the team but not by lowering their association with the team.

Finally, we were also interested in the possibility that the tendency for highly identified fans to exhibit proactive pessimism would manifested in their behavioral intentions to attend games. That is, will the proactive pessimism simply involve cognitive distortions (i.e., expectations for success), or will it also impact behavioral intentions (i.e., desire to attend games during the upcoming season)? Because past work (Sheppard et al., 1996) on proactive pessimism had focused on cognitive distortions (e.g., lowering expectations for success on a test) rather than on behavioral intentions (e.g., likelihood of taking another college course from a given professor), it was not feasible to offer specific hypotheses about proactive pessimism and behavioral intentions. Rather, this topic was examined within the framework of a research question examining whether or not the proactive pessimistic tendencies of highly identified fans would also be manifested in their desire to attend the target team's games.

METHOD

Participants and Design

The original sample consisted of 239 college student participants. However, 146 subjects failed to complete the Time 1 questionnaire, failed to complete the Time 2 questionnaire, and/or did not report having a favorite Major League Baseball team. Thus, these individuals were removed from the data set resulting in a final sample of 93 persons (39 males, 53 females, 1 not reporting). Participants earned extra course credit in their course in exchange for participation. They had a mean age of 20.90 years ($SD = 2.86$). The design for the study was a 2 (Level of Team Identification: High or Low) x 2 (Testing Session: Time 1 and Time 2) mixed factorial. The first variable was a grouping variable while the second variable was a repeated measures within-subjects variable.

Materials and Procedure

Time 1 session. The Time 1 session occurred approximately four weeks prior to the start of the Major League Baseball season (i.e., early March). Upon entering the Time 1 session and providing their consent, participants (tested in groups) were handed a questionnaire packet containing three sections. The first section contained three demographic items assessing age, gender, and the last four digits of the participant's social security number (this information was used to match the Time 1 and Time 2 questionnaires). The second section asked participants to list their favorite Major League Baseball team and to complete the Sport Spectator Identification Scale (SSIS; Wann and Branscombe, 1993) with this team as the target. The SSIS contains 7 Likert-scale items with response options ranging from 1 (low identification) to 8 (high identification). Thus, higher numbers represented greater levels of identification. The SSIS has been used in a number of studies involving sport fans and has strong reliability and validity (see Wann and Branscombe, 1993; Wann et al., 2001).

In the third section, participants completed a series of items designed to assess their expectations for and excitement about the upcoming season for the team they had targeted on the SSIS. First, participants were asked to indicate the likelihood that they would attend one of the team's home games during the upcoming season as well as the likelihood that they would attend one of the team's road games. These two items were Likert-scale in format and had response options ranging from 1 (not likely to attend) to 8 (very likely to attend). Participants were then asked five Likert-scale questions assessing their beliefs that the team would win their division, play in the World Series, win the World Series, how excited their were about the upcoming season, and how much they were looking forward to the upcoming season. These items were again scored on an eight-point scale ranging from 1 (not likely to win, not likely to play in, not excited, not looking forward to) to 8 (very likely to win, very likely to play in, very excited, very much looking forward to). Finally, subjects were asked to indicate if the team they had targeted on the SSIS was "my favorite sport team to follow." Response options to this Likert-scale item ranged from 1 (totally disagree) to 8 (totally agree). After completing the questionnaire packet (15 minutes), participants were debriefed, reminded that there would be a post-test session in the coming weeks, and excused from the testing session.

Time 2 session. The Time 2 session occurred approximately three weeks after the Time 1 session and one week prior to the start of the Major League Baseball season (i.e., very late March). Upon entering the session and providing their consent, participants (tested in groups) were handed a questionnaire packet nearly identical to that used in Time 1. The only difference was that the gender and age items were omitted from the post-test protocol. Thus, respondents were again asked to provide the last four digits of their social security number (for matching purposes), complete the SSIS for their favorite Major League Baseball team, and complete the items assessing expectations for and excitement about the upcoming season for the target team. After completing the Time 2 questionnaire (15 minutes), participants were debriefed and excused from the testing session.

RESULTS

Preliminary Analyses

Table 1. Names, Numbers, and Percentages of Major League Baseball Teams Listed as a Favorite

Team	Number Listing Team	Percentage Listing Team
St. Louis Cardinals	38	41
Atlanta Braves	16	17
Chicago Cubs	10	11
New York Yankees	8	9
Boston Red Sox	4	4
Cincinnati Reds	4	4
New York Mets	2	2
Philadelphia Phillies	2	2
Chicago White Sox	1	1
Detroit Tigers	1	1
Houston Astros	1	1
Los Angeles Dodgers	1	1
Milwaukee Brewers	1	1
Minnesota Twins	1	1
Oakland A's	1	1
Pittsburgh Pirates	1	1
San Francisco Giants	1	1

Participants listed 17 different Major League Baseball Teams as a favorite. The teams and percentages listed as a favorite appear in Table 1. The seven items comprising the Time 1 SSIS (Cronbach's alpha = .961) and the Time 2 SSIS (alpha = .959) were combined to form a single index of Time 1 identification and Time 2 identification. A median split procedure was performed on the Time 1 identification scores to establish a low identification group ($n = 45$, $M = 22.36$, $SD = 8.29$, range = 7 to 35) and a high identification group ($n = 48$, $M = 45.50$, $SD = 5.74$, range = 36 to 56). A one-way analysis of variance (ANOVA) indicated that the two groups were significantly different in their levels of identification with the favorite Major League Baseball team, $F(1, 91) = 247.72$, $p < .001$. The two attendance items (i.e., likelihood of attending a home game and a road game) were combined to form a single index of attendance likelihood for both the Time 1 (alpha = .658) and the Time 2 (alpha = .641) sessions. The five items assessing expectations for and excitement about the upcoming season for the target team were combined to form a single index of Time 1 evaluations (alpha = .92) and Time 2 evaluations (alpha = .91). Men and women did not significantly differ on any of the dependent measures at either Time 1 or at Time 2 (all Fs < 1.90, all ps > .15). Consequently, all subsequent analyses were conducted across gender.

Evaluation Measures and Team Identification

The two hypotheses and one research question were analyzed using a series of 2 (Level of Team Identification: high or low) x 2 (Testing Session: Time 1 and Time 2) mixed factorial ANOVAs (see Table 2 for all means and standard deviations). Hypothesis 1 predicted that highly identified fans would exhibit proactive pessimism as indicated by lowered team evaluations at Time 2, relative to Time 1. The 2 x 2 ANOVA computed on the Time 1 and Time 2 evaluation indices revealed a significant team identification main effect, $F(1, 91) = 59.47$, $p < .001$. As one would expect, averaged across time, highly identified fans gave more positive evaluations to their favorite Major League Baseball team ($M = 6.07$, $SD = 1.21$) than did lowly identified fans ($M = 3.83$, $SD = 1.58$). The analysis failed to reveal a significant time main effect as persons (across identification group) did not report differential team evaluations at Time 1 ($M = 5.00$, $SD = 1.86$) and Time 2 ($M = 4.97$, $SD = 1.80$), $F(1, 91) = 0.07$, $p > .75$. In support of Hypothesis 1, the two-way interaction was significant, $F(1, 91) = 7.06$, $p < .01$. As seen in Table 2, highly identified fans became more cautious in their evaluations of the team as the season approached. Indeed, a t-test revealed that the decrease in evaluations from Time 1 to Time 2 was significant for these persons, $t(47) = 2.60$, $p < .02$. Participants low in team identification did not report a significant change in evaluations from Time 1 to Time 2, $t(44) = -1.42$, $p > .15$.

Thus, Hypothesis 1 was supported as highly identified fans, but not those lower in identification, lowered their evaluations of their team as the season neared. However, such changes over time were not expected for the participants' psychological connection to their team.

Table 2. Means and Standard Deviations for the Dependent Measures by Level of Team Identification and Time

Measure	Low Identification		High Identification	
	Time 1	Time 2	Time 1	Time 2
Evaluation of team	3.74(1.56)	3.92(1.71)	6.18(1.25)	5.95(1.25)
Team identification	22.36(8.29)	22.40(9.51)	45.50(5.74)	44.35(6.78)
Target team is favorite	3.56(2.33)	3.22(2.10)	6.56(1.93)	6.31(1.75)
Likelihood of attendance	2.24(1.61)	2.54(1.88)	5.01(2.16)	4.77(2.14)

Note: Standard deviations appear in parentheses below each mean.

Specifically, Hypothesis 2 predicted that highly identified fans would not exhibit a Time 1 to Time 2 change in their association with the team, as assessed in two ways: via their level of team identification and via the extent to which the target team was their favorite sport team. The first 2 x 2 ANOVA, computed on the Time 1 and Time 2 identification scores, yielded a significant team identification main effect, $F(1, 91) = 231.51$, $p < .001$, indicating simply that, averaged across time, the highly identified participants ($M = 44.93$, $SD = 5.66$) had higher levels of identification than those with low levels of identification ($M = 22.38$, $SD = 8.44$). The time main effect was not statistically significant, $F(1, 91) = 0.90$, $p > .30$. As expected, the two-way interaction was also not significant, $F(1, 91) = 1.05$, $p > .30$. As detailed in Table 2, there was little change in identification scores from Time 1 to Time 2 for both identification groups. The second ANOVA, computed on the Time 1 and Time 2 "team is favorite" item, again yielded a significant team identification main effect, $F(1, 91) = 62.01$, $p < .001$, which logically indicated that, averaged across time, the highly identified participants ($M = 6.44$, $SD = 1.69$) were more likely to view the target team as a favorite than those with low levels of identification ($M = 3.39$, $SD = 2.04$). The time main effect was marginally significant, $F(1, 91) = 3.06$, $p = .08$. Once again, as expected and consistent with Hypothesis 2, the two-way interaction was not significant, $F(1, 91) = 0.06$, $p > .80$.

The final ANOVA investigated the research question probing whether or not the proactive pessimistic tendencies of highly identified fans would be manifested in their desire to attend the target team's games. As one would expect, the ANOVA yielded a significant team identification main effect, $F(1, 91) = 40.92$, $p < .001$, indicating that, averaged across time, highly identified participants ($M = 4.89$, $SD = 2.06$) had reported a greater likelihood of attending their team's games than did those with low levels of identification ($M = 2.39$, $SD = 1.67$). The time main effect was not statistically significant, $F(1, 91) = 0.07$, $p > .75$. The two-way interaction was significant, $F(1, 91) = 5.18$, $p < .05$. As indicated in Table 2, lowly identified participants reported an increased likelihood of attending their team's games at Time 2 while highly identified participants reported a decreased likelihood of attending their team's games. However, post hoc t-tests indicated that each of these individual findings were only marginally significant [lowly identified persons: $t(44) = -1.95$, $p = .06$; highly identified persons: $t(44) = 1.34$, $p = .18$].

DISCUSSION

It was hypothesized that sport fans would exhibit proactive pessimism by lowering their evaluations of their team's chances for a successful season as the season approached and that this pattern of effects would be most prominent among highly identified fans. We did not expect these same highly identified fans to report lowered levels of interest in the team. Thus, we expected highly identified fans to cope with the possibility that their team would perform poorly by lowering their expectations for the team but not by lowering their psychological connection to it. Indeed, the results confirmed this pattern of effects. Specifically, highly identified fans lowered their expectations for team success as the season approached (i.e., from Time 1 to Time 2). Low identified fans did not reported statistically significant Time 1 to Time 2 changes in team evaluations. With respect to psychological connection to the team, neither highly nor lowly identified persons reported Time 1 to Time 2 changes in either team identification as assessed by the SSIS (Wann and Branscombe, 1993) or in the extent that the team was perceived to be their favorite team. Thus, as a season approaches, highly identified fans cope by becoming more cautious in their expectations for team success (thus mirroring past work on the tendency for college students to lower their estimates of exam performance as the test draws near, Sheppard et al., 1996). They do not cope by lowering their associations with or interest in the team. Simply put, they still care as deeply about the team, they are just more reserved in their expectations of success, thereby proactively coping with a potential threat to their social identity (i.e., the team's potential poor play).

We were also interested in the possibility that highly identified fans would exhibit proactive pessimism in their attendance intentions. Analyses examining this research question revealed a significant two-way interaction in which lowly identified persons reported Time 1 to Time 2 increases in the likelihood that they would attend their team's games while the highly identified participants reported decreases. This suggests that the tendencies to engage in proactive pessimism among highly identified fans may be manifested behaviorally in their attendance decisions. For these persons, their interest in the team remained high, but their desire (as measured by reported likelihood) to attend decreased. This may indicate that, given their lowered expectations for the team, the highly identified fans may have been less excited about watching their team perform in person. This possibility has empirical support from numerous studies documented the positive relationship between team performance and attendance (e.g., Baade and Tiehen, 1990; Brooks, 1994; Zhang, Pease, Hui, and Michaud, 1995). For fans with low levels of identification, their increased desire to attend the team's games may have been a reflection of the excitement of the upcoming season. For these persons, there was no need to feel threatened by the team's potentially poor performance and hence, no need to engage in proactive pessimism. Consequently, they were more likely to exhibit increased interest in attending the team's games (the team's performances would not be viewed as a threat to their social identity).

However, it warrants mention that, although the proactive pessimism of highly identified fans was reflected in their attendance decisions, testing for this project occurred at a regional university located more than 200 miles from the nearest Major League team (the St. Louis Cardinals). Many of the teams listed (e.g., the Boston Red Sox, Los Angeles Dodgers, and San Francisco Giants) were more than 1,000 miles away. It is unclear what impact this may have had on answers to the items on attendance decisions. For many of the participants it would have been quite costly in terms of time, money, and effort to attended one of their team's games (but not unthinkable as indicated by the means reported in Table 2). Given that cost is a key variable in fans' decisions to attend games (Wann et al., 2001), it may well be that this level of effort and expense, combined with the tendency to use proactive pessimism, led to the attendance effects reported above. Future researchers should attempt to replicate these findings with attendance intentions for a local team (and, thus, attendance that would be far less costly). In addition, it seems plausible that one's behavioral intentions to attend a team's games will shift as a season progresses, given that the team's performance up to that point in time would serve as an objective measure of the team's success (and, hence, likelihood for continued success). Thus, the current investigation should be replicated during a season to see if fans continue to use proactive pessimism, if the use of this strategy impacts attendance intentions, and to explore how recent team performance (i.e., the team's record up to that point in the season) impacts the results.

Another line of future research may want to further examine the impact of threat on the use of proactive pessimism by manipulating the team's prognosis for the season. In the current investigation, no information about the teams' expected performances for the upcoming season was provided. Rather, the participants' expectations were their own. It would be interesting to manipulate expectations of performance by providing the subjects with an "expert" analysis of the team for the approaching season. By having some subjects read that the team should do very well (low threat) while others read that the team will likely struggle (high threat), one could very well find differences in the threat conditions. Specifically, one would expect an especially high use of proactive pessimism (i.e., large decreases in team evaluations as a season draws near) among highly identified fans who read that the team will likely perform poorly.

It is also important to compare the current set of findings with previously published reports on the biased recollections and predictions of team performance exhibited by highly identified fans (Dietz-Uhler and Murrell, 1999; Funk and James, 2001; Wann, 1994, 1996; Wann and Branscombe, 1993; Wann and Dolan, 1994b). This body of literature indicates that, compared to low identified fans, persons with higher levels of allegiance tend to be positively biased in their evaluations of the team's future performances (e.g., estimate greater numbers of victories). The current investigation found that, relative to less identified persons, highly identified fans decreased their evaluations of the team as a season approached. However, this finding is not contrary to the aforementioned literature on the biased evaluations. Rather, the bias of highly identified fans is simply less prominent as a season approaches. One would not expect the decrease to become so great as to lead highly identified fans to report lower evaluations than lowly identified individuals. Indeed, the Time 2 evaluations of highly identified were still much more positive than those of less identified fans. Rather, the gap in evaluations separating the two groups merely shrinks as the season draws near.

In closing, it should be noted that that data reported above replicate many previously documented findings among sport fans. For instance, the highly identified subjects reported more favorable evaluations of the team than did those low in team identification (see the ANOVA for Hypothesis 1). This finding replicates numerous studies on the biased evaluations of highly identified fans, relative to those with lower levels of allegiance (e.g., Wann and Dolan, 1994b). Further, the current investigation adds to the growing body of literature indicating that level of team identification is an extremely stable trait (see Wann, 1996, 2000; Wann et al., 1994). And finally, as indicated by the main effect on identification for attendance decisions, the current work mirrors a large body of literature indicating that level of team identification is a strong predictor attendance decisions (e.g., Wakefield and Sloan, 1995; Wann, Roberts, and Tindall, 1999; Williamson, Zhang, Pease, and Gaa, 2003).

REFERENCES

Baade, R. A., and Tiehen, L. J. (1990). An analysis of major league baseball attendance, 1969-1987. *Journal of Sport and Social Issues, 14*, 14-32.

Bat-Chava, Y. (1993). Group identification and self-esteem of deaf adults. *Personality and Social Psychology Bulletin, 20,* 494-502.

Bat-Chava, Y. (1994). Antecedents of self-esteem in deaf people: A meta-analytic review. *Rehabilitation Psychology, 38,* 221-234.

Branscombe, N. R., Ellemers, N., Spears, R., and Doosje, B. (1999). The context and content of social identity threat. In N. Ellemers, R. Spears, and B. Doosje (Eds.), *Social identity* (pp. 35-58). Oxford, UK: Blackwell.

Brooks, C. M. (1994*). Sport marketing: Competitive business strategies for sports.* Englewood Cliffs, NJ: Prentice-Hall.

Brown, B. B., and Lohr, N. (1987). Peer group affiliation and adolescent self-esteem: An integration of ego-identity and symbolic-interaction theories. *Journal of Personality and Social Psychology, 52,* 47-55.

Cohen, S., and Wills, T. A. (1985). Stress, social support, and the buffering hypothesis. *Psychological Bulletin, 98,* 310-357.

Compton, W. C. (2005). *An introduction to positive psychology.* Belmont, CA: Thomson Wadsworth.

Crocker, J., and Major, B. (1989). Social stigma and self-esteem: The self-protective properties of stigma. *Psychological Review, 96,* 608-630.

Diener, E., and Clifton, D. (2002). Life satisfaction and religiosity in broad probability samples. *Psychological Inquiry, 13,* 206-209.

Dietz-Uhler, B., and Murrell, A. (1999). Examining fan reactions to game outcomes: A longitudinal study of social identity. *Journal of Sport Behavior, 22,* 15-27.

Funk, D. C., and James, J. (2001). The psychological continuum model: A conceptual framework for understanding an individual's psychological connection to sport. *Sport Management Review, 4,* 119-150.

Hirt, E. R., Zillmann, D., Erickson, G. A., and Kennedy, C. (1992). Costs and benefits of allegiance: Changes in fans' self-ascribed competencies after team victory versus defeat. *Journal of Personality and Social Psychology, 63,* 724-738.

Hogg, M. A., and Abrams, D. (1990). Social motivation, self-esteem, and social identity. In D. Abrams and M. A. Hogg (Eds.), *Social identity theory: Constructive and critical advances* (pp. 28-47). New York: Harvester Wheatsheaf.

Linville, P. W. (1987). Self-complexity as a cognitive buffer against stress related illness and depression. *Journal of Personality and Social Psychology, 52,* 663-676.

Markman, K. D., and Hirt, E. R. (2002). Social prediction and the "allegiance bias." *Social Cognition, 20,* 58-86.

Melnick, M. J. (1993). Searching for sociability in the stands: A theory of sports spectating. *Journal of Sport Management, 7,* 44-60.

Ouwerkerk, J. W., Ellemers, N., and de Gilder, D. (1999). Group commitment and individual effort in experimental and organizational contexts. In N. Ellemers, R. Spears, and B. Doosje (Eds.), *Social identity* (pp. 184-204). Oxford, UK: Blackwell.

Rowe, J. W., and Kahn, R. L. (1998). *Successful aging.* New York: Dell.

Schwarz, N., Strack, F., Kommer, D., and Wagner, D. (1987). Soccer, rooms, and the quality of your life: Mood effects on judgments of satisfaction with life in general and with specific domains. *European Journal of Social Psychology, 17,* 69-79.

Shepperd, J. A., Ouellette, J. A., and Fernandez, J. K. (1996). Abandoning unrealistic optimism: Performance estimates and the temporal proximity of self-relevant feedback. *Journal of Personality and Social Psychology, 70,* 844-855.

Smith, G. J. (1988). The noble sports fan. *Journal of Sport and Social Issues, 12,* 54-65.

Spears, R., Doosje, B., and Ellemers, N. (1997). Self-stereotyping in the face of threats to group status and distinctiveness: The role of group identification. *Personality and Social Psychology Bulletin, 23,* 538-553.

Tykocinski, O. E., Pick, D., and Kedmi, D. (2002). Retroactive pessimism: A different kind of hindsight bias. *European Journal of Social Psychology, 32,* 577-588.

Wakefield, K. L., and Sloan, H. J. (1995). The effects of team loyalty and selected stadium factors on spectator attendance. *Journal of Sport Management, 9,* 153-172.

Wann, D. L. (in press). Understanding the positive social psychological benefits of sport team identification: The team identification – social psychological health model. *Group Dynamics: Theory, Research, and Practice.*

Wann, D. L. (1994). Biased evaluations of highly identified sport spectators: A response to Hirt and Ryalls. *Perceptual and Motor Skills, 79,* 105-106.

Wann, D. L. (1996). Seasonal changes in spectators' identification and involvement with and evaluations of college basketball and football teams. *The Psychological Record, 46,* 201-215.

Wann, D. L. (2000). Further exploration of seasonal changes in sport fan identification: Investigating the importance of fan expectations. *International Sport Journal, 4,* 119-123.

Wann, D. L., and Branscombe, N. R. (1993). Sports fans: Measuring degree of identification with the team. *International Journal of Sport Psychology, 24,* 1-17.

Wann, D. L., and Branscombe, N. R. (1995). Influence of identification with a sports team on objective knowledge and subjective beliefs. *International Journal of Sport Psychology, 26,* 551-567.

Wann, D. L., Dimmock, J. A., and Grove, J. R. (2003). Generalizing the team identification – psychological health model to a different sport and culture: The case of Australian Rules football. *Group Dynamics: Theory, Research, and Practice, 7,* 289-296.

Wann, D. L., and Dolan, T. J. (1994a). Attributions of highly identified sport spectators. *The Journal of Social Psychology, 134,* 783-792.

Wann, D. L., and Dolan, T. J. (1994b). Influence of spectators' identification on evaluation of the past present and future performance of a sports team. *Perceptual and Motor Skills, 78,* 547-552.

Wann, D. L., and Dolan, T. J. (1994c). Spectators' evaluations of rival and fellow fans. *The Psychological Record, 44,* 351-358.

Wann, D. L., Dolan, T. J., McGeorge, K. K., and Allison, J. A. (1994). Relationships between spectator identification and spectators' perceptions of influence, spectators' emotions, and competition outcome. *Journal of Sport and Exercise Psychology, 16,* 347-364.

Wann, D. L., and Grieve, F. G. (2005). Biased evaluations of ingroup and outgroup spectator behavior at sporting events: The importance of team identification and threats to social identity. *Journal of Social Psychology, 145,* 531-545.

Wann, D. L., and Grieve, F. G., and Martin, J. (2006). *Use of retroactive pessimism as a method of coping with identity threat: The impact of group identification.* Manuscript submitted for publication.

Wann, D. L., Friedman, K., McHale, M., and Jaffe, A. (2003). The Norelco Sport Fanatics Survey: Examining behaviors of sport fans. *Psychological Reports, 92,* 930-936.

Wann, D. L., Inman, S., Ensor, C. L., Gates, R. D., and Caldwell, D. S. (1999). Assessing the psychological well-being of sport fans using the Profile of Mood States: The importance of team identification. *International Sports Journal, 3,* 81-90.

Wann, D. L., Melnick, M. J., Russell, G. W., and Pease, D. G. (2001). *Sport fans: The psychology and social impact of spectators.* New York: Routledge Press.

Wann, D. L., and Pierce, S. (2005). The relationship between sport team identification and social well-being: Additional evidence supporting the team identification – social psychological health model. *North American Journal of Psychology, 7,* 117-124.

Wann, D. L., Roberts, A., and Tindall, J. (1999). The role of team performance, team identification, and self-esteem in sport spectators' game preferences. *Perceptual and Motor Skills, 89,* 945-950.

Wann, D. L., and Schrader, M. P. (2000). Controllability and stability in the self-serving attributions of sport spectators. *Journal of Social Psychology, 140,* 160-168.

Wann, D. L., Schrader, M. P., and Adamson, D. R. (1998). The cognitive and somatic anxiety of sport spectators. *Journal of Sport Behavior, 21,* 322-337.

Wann, D. L., and Wilson, A. M. (2001). The relationship between the sport team identification of basketball spectators and the number of attributions generated to explain a team's performance. *International Sports Journal, 5,* 43-50.

Williamson, D. P., Zhang, J. J., Pease, D. G., and Gaa, J. P. (2003). Dimensions of spectator identification associated with women's professional basketball game attendance. *International Journal of Sport Management, 4,* 59-91.

Zhang, J. J., Pease, D. G., Hui, S. C., and Michaud, T. J. (1995). Variables affecting the spectator decision to attend NBA games. *Sport Marketing Quarterly, 4*(4), 29-39.

Zillmann, D., Bryant, J., and Sapolsky, B. S. (1989). Enjoyment from sports spectatorship. In J. H. Goldstein (Ed.), *Sports, games, and play: Social and psychological viewpoints* (2nd ed., pp. 241-278). Hillsdale, NJ: Erlbaum.

In: Sports and Athletics Developments
Editor: James H. Humphrey, pp. 45-56

ISBN: 978-1-60456-205-7
© 2008 Nova Science Publishers, Inc.

Chapter 3

SPORTS SPECTATOR BEHAVIOR FOR COLLEGIATE WOMEN'S BASKETBALL

Jennifer Y. Mak[*], *Anita N. Lee*[**] *and Juliet Donahue*[*]
[*]Marshall University
[**]Plymouth State University

ABSTRACT

The purpose of this study was to examine the relationships between the Desire to attend collegiate women's basketball (DES) and three aspects of attending collegiate women's basketball games. The participants were spectators of a National Collegiate Athletic Association (NCAA) Division I women's basketball game ranging in age from 18 to 70 ($N = 312$). The Modified Sports Consumers Questionnaire (Milne & McDonald, 1999) was administered during a basketball game. After exploratory factor analysis (EFA) and confirmatory factor analysis (CFA), three factors (Habit, Attitude, and Satisfaction) with 19 items were retained for Sports Spectator Behavior (SSB). Structural equation modeling was used to analyze the relationships among DES and three SSB factors. The findings revealed that the DES was positively related to the Habit of affiliating themselves with sports (HAB) and the Attitude toward watching sports (ATT), but negatively related to the Satisfaction of watching sports (SAT). The three main predictors of SSB account for 85% of the variance of DES.

Spectator behavior is always a major concern of sports organizers. An understanding of sports spectator behavior allows sports managers to promote programs effectively. Numerous researchers have tried to assess sports spectator behavior in specific sports settings such as the Women's National Basketball Association and the National Basketball Association (Williamson, Zhang, Pease, & Gaa, 2003; Zhang, Connaughton, & Vaughn, 2004; Zhang & Pease, 2001; Zhang, Pease, Hui, & Michaud, 1995; Zhang et al., 2003; Zhang, Piatt, Ostroff, & Wright 2005; Zhang & Smith, 1997; Zhang, Wall, & Smith, 2000), the Japanese Professional Soccer League (Mahony, Nakazawa, Funk, James, & Gladden, 2002), collegiate football (Kahle, Kambara, & Rose, 1996; Swanson, Gwinner, Larson, & Janda, 2003), professional sports (Roy & Graeff 2003), and men's and/or women's collegiate basketball (Fink, Trail, & Anderson 2002; Trail, Anderson, & Fink, 2002, 2005; Trail, Fink, & Anderson, 2003). Collegiate women's basketball, meanwhile, has always been overlooked. With the continual increase in number of spectators attending collegiate women's basketball games, the investigation of sports spectator behavior for collegiate women's basketball becomes necessary. This study aims to examine the relationships between the Desire to attend collegiate women's basketball (DES) and three aspects of Sports Spectator Behavior (SSB): (a) Habit of affiliating themselves with sports (HAB), (b) Attitude toward watching sports (ATT), and (c) Satisfaction of watching sports (SAT). As an exploratory study, the present study should allow sports-related personnel to have a better understanding of spectator behavior for collegiate women's basketball.

Since the passage of Title IX of the Education Amendment of 1972, female sports participation has increased. (Carpenter & Acosta, 2006; Coakley, 2003; Mahony & Pastore, 1998; Mak, 2006). The number of female high school athletes has increased from 7.4% ($n = 294,015$) to 41.5% ($n = 2,784,154$) between 1971-72 to 2000-01, and female college athletes have increased from 15.0% ($n = 29,972$) to 42.0% ($n = 150,916$) in the same 30 year period (Mak, 2006; National Collegiate Athletic Association, 2002; National Federation of State High School Associations, 2001). Accordingly, the numbers of spectators at women's professional and amateur sports events have been increasing steadily (Coakley, 2003; Funk, Mahony, & Ridinger, 2002; Lough, 1996). Particularly, the number of spectators in women's basketball continues to increase at both collegiate and professional levels (Fink et al., 2002).

Researches have shown that differences exist between fans of men's basketball teams and fans of women's basketball teams (Fink et al., 2002; Kahle, Duncan, Dalaka, & Aiken, 2001). Fink et al. (2002) found that: (a) spectators in women's games exhibited greater influence by promotions, family, friends, and ticket pricing than spectators in male's games; (b) spectators in male's games reported stronger sentiment regarding team media and team merchandise; and (c) spectators in women's games were more loyal than spectators in male's games.

Fink et al. (2002) admitted that "little marketing research is done within intercollegiate athletic programs; as a result, those programs are unable to effectively segment current and potential markets. Often, women's teams are "marketed" in the same manner as men's teams – if at all" (p. 9). Brennan (2001) acknowledged that "I think women's team sports in particular have uncovered what I call an emerging fan" (p. 3C). So, it is critical for sports marketers to identify the factors affecting attendance at women's basketball games. More research on sports spectator behavior for collegiate women's basketball needs to be conducted in order to close this gap.

METHODOLOGY

Participants

Participants (N = 312) for the current study included males (n = 132) and females (n = 173). Seven participants did not report their gender. The participants were spectators at a collegiate women's basketball game from a National Collegiate Athletic Association (NCAA) Division I institution in the mid-Atlantic region.

Measuring Instruments and Procedures

A modified version of the spectator typology for sports spectator behavior (Milne & McDonald, 1999) was used to measure the domain of motivational constructs applicable to sports spectatorship. Spectators aged 18 and above were asked to complete the questionnaire before or during the half–time break of an NCAA Division I women's basketball game. Questionnaires were distributed at all the entrances and in each section of the arena.

Statistical Analyses

An analysis of frequency distribution was used to describe the demographic information of the participants. The Cronbach Alpha Coefficient was used to test the reliability and internal consistency of the questionnaire. Exploratory factor analysis (EFA) and confirmatory factor analysis (CFA) were utilized to analyze the factorial validity of the factors on the instrument. Structural equation modeling (SEM) analysis was used to assess the proposed structural model as shown in Figure 1.

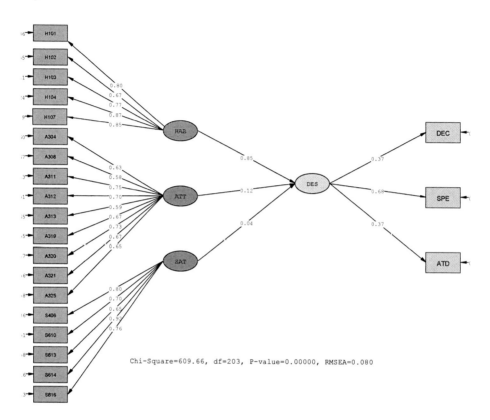

Figure 1. Proposed Structural Model.

The Bollen and Long (1993) five-step procedure (model specification, identification, estimation, testing goodness-of-fit statistics, and respecification) was used in the SEM analysis. The latent variable of DES was considered as an exogenous variable. The subscales of SSB including Habit, Attitude, and Satisfaction were the endogenous variables when testing the proposed structural model. The PRELIS 2.30 and LISREL 8.30 programs were utilized. The PRELIS 2.30 program was used to test for multivariate normality, and to obtain the variance/covariance matrix. The assessment of model fit was based on the results of the root-mean-square error of approximation (RMSEA), the comparative fit index (CFI), the standardized root mean square residual (SRMR), and the Chi-square ratio. The RMSEA is an absolute noncentrality based fit index to assess how well the model approximates the data by determining the lack of fit of the model to the population covariance matrix, expressed as the discrepancy per degree of freedom. An RMSEA value of .05 or less generally indicates a close fit, a value up to .08 indicates a fair fit, while a value over .10 indicates an unacceptable fit (Browne & Cudeck, 1993). CFI had a range of zero to 1. A CFI cutoff value close to .95 or higher indicates a close fit, and values up to .90 indicates a reasonable fit (Hu & Bentler, 1999). The SRMR is the average difference between the sample variances and co-variances. Similarly, the SRMR has a range of zero to 1.00. Good-fitting models have a small SRMR. A value of .05 or less is desired and a value up to .08 indicates a reasonable fit (Hu & Bentler, 1999). Hatcher (1994) suggested that a ratio of less than 2.00 would be desirable for the ratio of Chi-square to the degree of freedom. A value close to 1 indicates a good fit and values between 2 to 5 indicate an acceptable fit (Jöreskog, 1969).

RESULTS

A total of 312 usable responses—which consisted of 132 males and 173 females, with the majority of Caucasian (89.3%) and with age range from 18 to 70—were collected from a Mid-Atlantic university. After EFA and CFA, three factors (HAB, ATT and SAT) with 19 items were retained in the SSB. The means of the 19 endogenous variables ranged from 2.71 to 4.40 with standard deviations ranged from .82 to 1.29 (see Table 1).

Various fit statistics were tested to provide information on the data model fit. The overall fit of the proposed structural model appeared to be poor (see Table 2). The goodness-of-fit index CFI did not reach the cut-off point of .90. Moreover, the RMSEA value was .080, which represented only a fair fit. The χ^2/df ratio was 3.00, which was higher than the desirable level of 2.00. The SRMR was .067, which indicated a reasonable fit (see Table 2). Therefore, the proposed structural model was rejected. According to Jöreskog and Sörbom (1996), improvement in fit is measured by a reduction in χ^2, which is expected to equal the modification index. After considering the results of the modification index, the decision was made to eliminate H101, H103, A311, A312, A313, A321, and S614 from the proposed structural model to form the alternative structural model (see Figure 2).

Table 1. Descriptive Information of 19 Observed Variables

Questions	Variables Code	Mean[1]	SD
Habit of affiliating themselves with Sports			
Watch sports events on television	H101	4.238	0.8186
Listen to sports on the radio	H102	3.049	1.2934
Read the sports pages of the newspaper	H103	4.277	1.1315
Watch or listen to sports news on television or radio	H104	4.396	0.9312
Talk about sports with your friends	H107	4.233	0.9509
Attitude toward watching sports			
Watching my favorite sports helps me develop a competitive ethic	A304	3.651	1.0410
Watching my favorite sports with group leads to improved social relationships	A308	3.852	0.9324
Enjoyment is enhanced by knowing the high degree of skill required to attain positive results	A311	4.095	0.8753
Enjoy watching highly skilled player perform	A312	4.337	0.8742
Enjoy watching because it is a difficult sport to master	A313	3.536	1.1671
Camaraderie among the people I watch with	A319	3.921	0.9003
Sports can be beautiful to watch	A320	4.112	0.9076
Enjoy watching the artistry	A321	4.059	0.8467
Watching has helped teach me the value of hard work and dedication	A325	4.060	0.9264
Satisfaction of watching sports			
Help me to reach my potential as an individual	S406	2.850	1.1373
Improved fitness /health	S610	3.495	1.1611
Enjoyment of risk-taking	S613	2.709	1.1635
Help me grow as a person	S614	3.102	1.1716
Sense of personal pride	S616	3.576	1.1120

[1]Mean scores were based on a 6-point Likert scale with the following options: "6" -- strongly agree; "5" – agree; "4" – slightly agree; "3" – slightly disagree; "2" – disagree; and "1" – strongly disagree.

The components and the overall fit of the alternative structural model are listed in Table 2. The alternative structural model RMSEA was .057, SRMR was .055 and

CFI was .95. The minimum fit function Chi-square value was 170.10 (df = 84, $p <$ .00). The Chi-square ratio was 2.03. The alternative structural model is considered to be a good fit. The SSB contained 12 items in the SSB with the Cronbach's alpha coefficient of each construct ranged from .71 to .76 and with an overall alpha coefficient of .81, indicating that the instrument was internally consistent and reliable.

Table 2. Goodness-of-Fit Indices of Structural Model

Model	χ^2	df	χ^2/df	RMSEA	SRMR	CFI	ECVI
Proposed Structural Model (19 items)	609.66	203	3.00	.080	.067	.87	2.28
Alterative Structural Model (12 items)	170.10	84	2.03	.057	.055	.95	.78

Note. RMSEA = Root Mean Square Error of Approximation; SRMR = Standardized Root Mean Square Residual; CFI = Comparative Fit Index; ECVI = Expected Cross-validation Index.

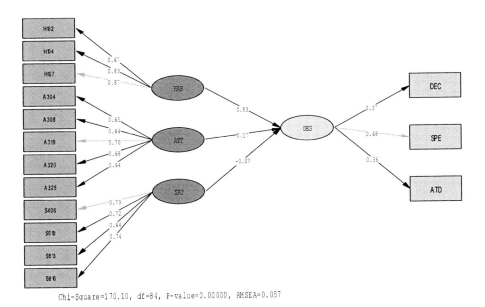

Chi-Square=170.10, df=84, P-value=0.00000, RMSEA=0.057

Figure 2. Alternative Structural Model.

The Desire to attend collegiate women's basketball games (DES) was positively related to the Habit of affiliating themselves with sports (HAB) and the Attitude toward watching sports (ATT), but negatively related to the Satisfaction of watching sports (SAT). Therefore, the more the participants affiliate themselves with sports and the more positive their attitude toward watching sports, the higher the desire to watch collegiate women's basketball games. The direct effect from HAB to DES ($\gamma = .83$) was significantly ($p < .05$) different from zero. The direct effect from ATT to DES ($\gamma = .17$) and SAT to DES ($\gamma = -.07$) were not significantly ($p > .05$) different from zero. The Lambda X values of the SSB indicators represented a high degree of validity with the range from .64 to .87. The strongest indicator for HAB is H107 ($\Lambda = .87$) (i.e. talk about sports with your friends). The strongest indicator for ATT is A319 ($\Lambda = .70$) (i.e. camaraderie among the people I watch my favorite sports with). The strongest indicator for SAT is S406 ($\Lambda = .79$) (i.e. helps me to reach my potential as an individual). The strongest predictor of DES is HAB ($\gamma = .83$), followed by ATT ($\gamma = .17$) and SAT ($\gamma = -.07$). In combination, the three predictors accounted for 85% of the variance of DES. The results supported that the SSB can be directly applied in predicting the desire to attend collegiate women's basketball games.

The Lambda Y values of the DES indicators ranged from .36 to .68. The strongest indicator is SPE ($\gamma = .68$) (i.e. interested in sports as a spectator), followed by DEC ($\gamma = .37$) (i.e. when to make decision to attend the collegiate women's basketball game) and ATD ($\gamma = .36$) (i.e. number of games attended in the past two years). The direct effects of SPE, DEC, and ATD were significantly ($p < .05$) different from zero. In the alternative model, SPE, DEC, and ATD exhibited positive relationships with DES.

CONCLUSION AND DISCUSSION

In the present study, the researchers found that the more the spectators affiliate themselves with sports, and the more positive their attitude toward watching sports, the higher the desire for the spectators to watch collegiate women's basketball games. In contrast, the higher the level of satisfaction of watching sports the spectators have, the lower the desire for the spectators to watch collegiate women's basketball games.

Regarding the Habit of the spectators to affiliate themselves with sports (HAB), talking about sports with friends and watching or listening to sports news on television or radio are the two key influencing factors. Whether sports spectators plan to attend collegiate women's basketball games or not, the decisions are mainly based on their habit of affiliating themselves with sports. In relation to the Attitude toward watching sports (ATT), the spectators perceived watching sports can help them to develop a competitive ethic and improve social relationships. Spectators value hard work, dedication, and beauty when they watch sports. The Satisfaction from watching sports (SAT) includes a sense of personal pride and an enjoyment of risk-taking. Spectators also perceived that watching sports could help them to reach their potential and improve their health and fitness.

The belief that watching sports enhances fitness and health levels is more of an illusion than a truth. Indeed, sports events provide a platform for sports spectators' dreams: sports allow spectators to be affiliated with and to observe risk-taking in an almost a risk-free environment. The assistance of sports marketers is suggested when planning for events, to ensure the collegiate women's basketball games can provide an effective platform to satisfy the sports spectators.

The researchers found that the factors influence individual to attend collegiate women's basketball games includes enjoyment of spectatorship, timeframe in deciding whether to attend a game, and past spectator experiences. In order to effectively market collegiate women's basketball games, sports marketers are encouraged to promote games to individuals who enjoy spectatorship, make an extra effort to retain past attendants, and focus the promotion to within less than a week before the game.

Further investigation of the relationship on sports spectator behavior for collegiate women's basketball and other women's collegiate sports should be conducted by recruiting participants from more than one institution. More participants recruited from different periods over the season should also be included in future studies.

REFERENCES

Bollen, K. A., & Long, J. S. (1993). *Testing structural equation models*. London: Sage.

Brennan C. (2001, May 8). Talking about revolution. *USA Today*, p. C3.

Browne, M. W., & Cudeck, R. (1993). Alternative ways of assessing model fit. In K. A. Bollen & J. S. Long (Eds.), *Testing structural equation models* (pp. 136-162). Newbury Park, CA: Sage.

Carpenter, L. J., & Acosta, V. (2006). *Women in intercollegiate sport: A longitudinal, national study twenty nine year update, 1977-2006.* Retrieved October 1, 2006, from Women in Sport/Title IX Web site: http://webpages.charter.net/womeninsport/AC_29YearStudy.pdf.

Coakley, J. (2003). *Sport in society: Issues and controversies* (8th ed.) New York: McGraw-Hill.

Fink, J. S., Trail, G. T., & Anderson, D. F. (2002). Environment factors associated with spectator attendance and sport consumption behavior: Gender and team differences. *Sport Marketing Quarterly, 11*(1), 8-19.

Funk, D. C., Mahony, D. F., & Ridinger, L. L. (2002).Characterizing consumer motivation as individual difference factors: Augmenting the Sport Interest Inventory (SII) to explain level of spectator support. *Sport Marketing Quarterly, 11*(1), 33-43.

Hatcher, L. (1994). *A step-by-step approach to using the SAS system for factor analysis and structural equation modeling.* Cary, NC: SAS Institute Inc.

Hu, L. T., & Bentler, P. (1999). Cutoff criteria for fit indexes in covariance structure analysis: Conventional criteria versus new alternatives. *Structural Equation Modeling, 6,* 1-55.

Jöreskog, K. G. (1969). A general approach to confirmatory maximum likelihood factor analysis. *Psychometrika, 34,* 183-202.

Jöreskog, K. & Sörbom, D. (1996). *LISREL 8: User's reference guide.* Chicago, IL: Scientific Software International, Inc.

Kahle, L., Duncan, M., Dalaka, V., & Aiken, D. (2001). The social values of fans for men's versus women's university basketball. *Sports Marketing Quarterly, 10*(2), 156-162.

Kahle, L. R., Kambara, K. M., & Rose, G. M. (1996). A functional model of fan attendance, motivations for college football. *Sport Marketing Quarterly, 5*(4), 51-60.

Lough, N. L. (1996). Factors affecting corporate sponsorship of women's sports. *Sports Marketing Quarterly, 5*(2), 11-20.

Mahony, D. F., Nakazawa, M., Funk, D. C., James, J. D., & Gladden, J. M. (2002). Motivational factors influencing the behavior of J. League spectators. *Sport Management Review, 5,* 1-24.

Mahony, D. F., & Pastore, D. (1998). Distributive justice: An examination of participation opportunities, revenues, and expenses at NCAA institutions—1973-1993. *Journal of Sport and Social Issues, 22,* 127-148.

Mak, J. Y. (2006). The impact of Title IX on athletics development in the United States. *Journal of Physical Education and Recreation (Hong Kong), 12*(1), 34-38.

Milne, G. R., & McDonald, M. A. (1999). *Sport marketing: Managing the exchange process.* Sudbury, MA: Jones and Bartlett.

National Collegiate Athletic Association. (2002, February). *1982-2001 NCAA sports sponsorship and participation report.* Retrieved October 15, 2006, from National Collegiate Athletic Association Web site: http://www.ncaa.org/library/research/participation_rates/1982-2001/index.html

National Federation of State High School Associations. (2001). *Athletics participation totals: Fact sheet.* Indianapolis, IN: Author.

Roy, D. P., & Graeff, T. R. (2003). Consumer attitudes toward cause-related marketing activities in professional sports. *Sport Marketing Quarterly, 12*(3), 163-172.

Swanson, S., Gwinner, K., Larson, B. V, & Janda, S. (2003), Motivations of college student game attendance and word-of-mouth behavior: The impact of gender differences. *Sport Marketing Quarterly, 12*(3), 151-162.

Trail, G. T., Anderson, D. F., & Fink, J. S. (2002). Examination of gender differences in importance of and satisfaction with venue factors at intercollegiate basketball games. *International Sports Journal, 6*, 51-64.

Trail, G. T., Anderson, D. F., & Fink, J. S. (2005). Consumer satisfaction and identity theory: A model of sport spectator conative loyalty. *Sport Marketing Quarterly, 14*(2), 98-111.

Trail, G. T., Fink, J. S., & Anderson, D. F. (2003). Sport spectator consumption behavior. *Sport Marketing Quarterly, 12*(1), 8-17.

Williamson, D. P., Zhang, J. J., Pease, D. G., & Gaa, J. P. (2003). Dimensions of spectator identification associated with women's professional basketball game attendance. *International Journal of Sport Management, 4*(1), 59-91.

Zhang, J. J., Connaughton, D. P., & Vaughn, C. (2004). The quality of special programs and services for NBA season ticket holders and their predictability to game consumption. *International Journal of Sport Marketing and Sponsorship, 6*(2), 99-116.

Zhang, J. J., & Pease, D. G. (2001). Socio-motivational factors affecting spectator attendance at professional basketball games. *International Journal of Sport Management, 2*(1), 31-59.

Zhang, J. J., Pease, D. G., & Hui, S. C. (1996). Value dimensions of professional sport as viewed by spectators. *Journal of Sport and Social Issues, 21*, 78-94.

Zhang, J. J., Pease, D. G., Hui, S. C., & Michaud, T. J. (1995). Variables affecting the spectator decision to attend NBA games. *Sport Marketing Quarterly, 4*(4), 29-39.

Zhang, J. J., Pennington-Gray, L., Connaughton, D. P., Braunstein, J. R, Ellis, M. H., Lam, E. T. C., et al. (2003). Understanding women's professional basketball game spectators: Sociodemographics, game consumption, and entertainment options. *Sport Marketing Quarterly, 12*(4), 228-243.

Zhang, J. J., Piatt, D. M., Ostroff, D. H., & Wright, J. W. (2005). Importance of in-game entertainment amenities at professional sporting events: A case for NBA season ticket holders. *Journal of Contemporary Athletics, 2*(1), 1-24.

Zhang, J. J., & Smith, D. W. (1997). Impact of broadcasting on the attendance of professional basketball games. *Sport Marketing Quarterly, 6*(1), 23-29.

Zhang, J. J., Wall, K. A., & Smith, D. W. (2000). To go or not? Relationship of selected variables to game attendance of professional basketball season ticket holders. *International Journal of Sport Management, 1*(3), 200-226.

In: Sports and Athletics Developments
Editor: James H. Humphrey, pp. 57-80

ISBN: 978-1-60456-205-7
© 2008 Nova Science Publishers, Inc.

Chapter 4

FUTURE PREDICTIONS OF DIVISION II ATHLETICS: TRENDS, ISSUES, AND EVENTS THAT MAY OCCUR IN THE UPCOMING DECADE

Thomas J. Aicher and Michael Sagas
Texas A and M University

ABSTRACT

The purpose of this study was to review previous prediction research in intercollegiate athletics, identify future trends in Division II Athletics, and compare predominately white colleges and universities (PWCU) to historically black colleges and universities (HBCU). Similar to previous research, this study utilized a modified Delphi technique to elicit responses from Athletic Directors and Senior Women Administrators of Division II level institutions. A total of 15 Athletic Directors and Senior Women Administrators responded to the first round of questionnaires and 29 in the second round. In all, 17 items were identified by the panelist in the areas of academics, NCAA governance, amateurism, gender equity, and financial conditions. The questionnaire further asked the respondents to indicate when the items may occur, the level of desirability of the item and impact that the item would have, and descriptive statistics were utilized to notate the average levels, and any anecdotal differences between HBCUs and PWCUs.

In 1993, the *Final Report of the Knight Commission on Intercollegiate Athletics* marked the beginning of the reform movement in intercollegiate athletics. Clifton R. Wharton, recently appointed co-chair of the Knight's Commission said "we are at a time when the lines between collegiate and professional sports are being blurred as never before" (NCAA News, 2006). With the proliferation of issues such as player stipends, gambling, corporate sponsorships, the continuation of the "arms race" and legal/organizational compliance, the athletic director position had to evolve. Athletic directors have many roles; they are educators, business people, police officers, marketers, public relation specialists, fund raisers, accountants, and must also have a working knowledge of legal and medical management issues (Geist and Pastore, 2002).

Significant changes in the structure and environment of intercollegiate athletics, and the attempts of many athletic departments to gain better control over their resources are reasons that athletic administrators need to gain a better understanding of the issues and trends that are going to occur in intercollegiate athletics. This insight will allow athletic directors the opportunity to strategically plan for the issues that they may face, and work towards trends that will be beneficial to their future. Secondly, some have mentioned that the issues faced by intercollegiate athletics are cyclical (Pastore and Schneider, 2004), so having predictions of the future and an understanding of the past will allow athletic administrators to predict cycles and prevent negative ones from occurring.

This study has three main purposes. First, to review previous research that has identified predictions of intercollegiate athletics in the future, second to identify trends and issues that will be faced by Division II athletic departments in particular, and lastly, compare the results of predominately white institutions to historically black colleges and universities. Research has been conducted at the Division I-A and I-AA level; however, no research has studied future predictions of Division II athletics. Given the larger dependency of Division II athletic programs on the university and the reduced revenue generation of Division II sports, funding may be one of the most important findings of this research. Different types of resolutions may precipitate through this study and prove to be beneficial to different athletic departments.

UNIQUE ASPECTS OF DIVISION II SCHOOLS

Division II athletics are an interesting sample to study in terms of future predictions in that they seem to be the forgotten Division in terms of research. Division II athletic departments are similar in structure to Division I, but due to the financial differences between the two divisions, Division II schools have to be more creative in their thinking. Division II athletic programs that compete in football operate at a greater deficit ($1,300,000), excluding Institutional support, than their Division counterparts without football ($1,100,000) (Fulks, 2001). In a study of Division I institutions, Agthe and Billings, (2000), posit a direct correlation between a profitable football team and Title IX compliance and that if a football team is non-profitable it will exacerbate gender inequity. With the lack of profits in Division II athletics, Title IX compliance among other issues should arise to a higher level than that found in studies of Division I and I-AA institutions.

Division II athletic programs must sponsor at least five sports for men and five sports for women (or four for men and six for women); whereas, Division I schools must have at least seven for men and women (or six for men and eight for women). In regards to attendance there are no minimum attendance figures for basketball and football as there are with Division I institutions. However, there are contest minimums and scheduling criteria (50% of their competitions must be with Division I-A or Division II schools) that they must adhere to similar to that of Division I schools.

There are a maximum number of scholarships that Division II institutions can provide to student athletes and in each sport are far less that that of their Division I counterparts. The make-up of the student body is normally compromised of in-state residents, especially in terms of the student athlete, and many of these students provide their own funding for the secondary education through grants, student loans and employment.

UNIQUE ASPECTS OF HISTORICALLY BLACK COLLEGES AND UNIVERSITIES

According to the U.S. Department of education, there are 228,000 students enrolled in 107 post secondary HBCUs and these schools are very unique in comparison to other post secondary institutions which make this group a unique interest of study. All HBCUs were founded before 1964, have an enrollment of more than 50% African-Americans, and concentrate on the education and uplifting of African-American Students (Brown and Davis, 2001). Similar to other post secondary schools, HBCUs vary by size, curriculum, and type such as public, private, two-year, or four-year institutions (Brown and Davis, 2001).

When it comes to athletics, HBCUs have a long standing history of spectator support and must utilize a competitive platform if they are able to survive in intercollegiate athletics at the Division I-AA or Division II level (Jackson, Lyons, and Gooden, 2001). Nance (1993) posits that black college sports create an event-style atmosphere that captures HBCU campuses, and because of their affordability offer a unique and entertaining experience for a good price. Athletic departments at HBCUs are challenged by many of the same issues that are raised by the Knight Commission, but are exacerbated because of the overwhelming financial pitfalls associated with competing at lower levels (Goss et. al, 2004). Jackson et. al (2001) concludes that HBCU athletic programs have smaller support staffs, low budgets (very low in comparison to other Division I and II schools) and lack expertise among personnel. This makes for an interesting group to study because they potentially have more issues to overcome than the average predominantly white college or university (PWCU).

Recently, HBCU conferences made a deal with Russell Athletic that will allow the company exclusive apparel licensing rights and in return will provide uniforms, performance apparel, casual apparel and athletic equipment to men's and women's basketball, soccer, football, baseball softball and volleyball teams (Bynum, 2004). This deal will provide HBCUs with much needed financial boost, but has created an environment in which the different institutions have joined forces to increase the bargaining power in the marketplace (Bynum, 2004). The new developments among HBCU in marketing, competition and their structure add to uniqueness of the group to be studied. HBCUs account for 30 of the 282 schools that compete at the Division II level and compete in men's and women's basketball, tennis, golf, cross country, indoor and outdoor track, volleyball, men's baseball soccer and football and women's bowling and softball (Sports ,2006). This study will attempt to ascertain any differences between HBCUs and PWCUs.

PREDICTING ISSUES AND TRENDS IN ATHLETICS

There is a dearth of research when predicting future issues that will be faced by intercollegiate athletics and the implications that the issues may have. A handful of studies have attempted to ascertain the future and past predictions of intercollegiate athletics (Krupa and Dunnavant ,1989; Branch and Crow, 1994; Drain and Ashley, 2000; Pastore and Schneider, 2004), but only one has looked at trends at HBCUs (Goss, Crow, Ashley and Jubenville, 2004). Each of the studies defined trends and issues in academics, amateurism, gender equity, NCAA governance, and financial conditions. This research assisted athletic administrators in identifying key issues and trends to focus their efforts on to ensure the stability and future growth of intercollegiate athletics. However, the research conducted has only looked at future predictions of Division I or Division I-AA schools, which leaves a significant portion of intercollegiate athletics unrepresented.

Krupa and Dunnavant (1989) the first to take a look into this topic by predicting events that would occur during the 1990's. Predictions were made in the areas of budget, integrity and reform, many of the major issues that the NCAA faced in the 1980's. These predictions were made based on a literature review; whereas, the remaining studies each utilized the Delphi technique to capture the opinions of the athletic directors in the context that they were studying.

Branch and Crow (1994) compiled the first list of issues that Division I athletic directors thought they may face in the next ten years. The study was conducted and utilized a modified Delphi technique to retain 8 respondents through two rounds (Branch and Crow, 1994). The original questionnaire was created through a literature review and the respondents were asked to make predictions of when the event would occur, the desirability of the event occurring and the impact that the event would have on intercollegiate athletics (Branch and Crow, 1994).

Drain and Ashley (2000) continued to study Division I Athletic Directors and their predictions of the issues that would be faced by intercollegiate athletics, the desirability and the impact that the event would have. A panel of 13 athletic directors was created and they were mailed a questionnaire that asked them to list the 10 most critical issues that Division I-A will face in the next 15 years (Drain and Ashley, 2000). After compiling the results of the first round a second questionnaire was sent out to the respondents and they were asked simply to agree or disagree that the issues listed were critical issues that athletic directors would face in the next 10 – 15 years. The final stages asked the respondents to rank the issues in order of importance and if statistically necessary they may have been asked to rank their responses again (Drain and Ashley, 2000).

Goss et. al (2000) utilized the modified Delphi technique; however, the population and study sample were Division I-AA HBCU athletic directors. With a total population of 15, no sampling method was used and one limitation of the study is that only 4 out of the 15 athletic directors responded (Goss et. al, 2004). The study utilized the initial results of Branch and Crow (1994), to create their second survey and similar to Branch and Crow (1994) asked respondents to predict when the event would occur, the desirability of the event and the impact that the event would have on intercollegiate athletics.

Each of the previous studies attempted to gain an understanding of the events that would occur in amateurism, academics, gender equity, NCAA governance and funding issues. The following sections give a review of their findings and posit reasons that each of these topics are integral to the future of intercollegiate athletics.

Academics. Over the past few years, academics have moved to the forefront of intercollegiate athletics. In 2004, the National Collegiate Athletic Association (NCAA) developed the Academic Progress Rate (APR) to determine the academic success of individual universities. A score of 925 becomes the cutoff point for each individual sport, meaning that teams that fall below the cut score are penalized accordingly. The first two year report was announced in 2006 showing that 15.4% of Division I teams were below the cut point, 24.1% men's and 8.0% women's (APR Statistics, 2006). The addition of this new reform supports previous study results that academic standards would be strengthened, but may lead to further concerns for the future of intercollegiate athletics.

Branch and Crow (1994) originally indicated that academic standards for admissions would be strengthened and proposition 42 would be passed with in the next ten years. Proposition 42 was passed shortly after the conclusion of the research and academic standards have been increased. Krupa and Dunnavant (1989) forecasted that academic standards for incoming freshman would be increased to closer meet the admission standards for the general student body. These are both supported by continuous research in that athletic directors feel that there will be more involvement of athletic departments in the educational mission of the institution (Drain and Ashley, 2000; Goss et. al, 2004) and the student athletes will be admitted under the same standards of other incoming students (Drain and Ashley, 2000; Goss et. al, 2004). Graduation rates have become more and more relevant with the creation of the APR and past research indicated the student athletes would compare favorably to that of the general student population (Drain and Ashley, 2004; Goss et. al, 2004).

Amateurism. In 2001, Division II changed its amateurism philosophy by eliminating the restriction that prospective student athletes could not receive prior payments for competing, they would now lose one year of eligibility for every year they competed (Pickle, 2005). Though the study may be considered out of date, Leonard (1986) surveyed 505 Division I, II, and III athletes and found that 60% of them felt reasonably compensated for their performance on the field. More recent research has indicated a growing number of student-athletes, coaches and university president interested in the outright payment to student athletes (Sage, 1998). However, Schneider (2000) suggests that student-athletes feel that they are inadequately compensated for their time and effort.

Continuous discussions, debates and research have led to similar results of the pros and cons of paying student-athletes (Schneider, 2000). Sage (1998) posits that student-athletes generate a tremendous amount of income for the university; Sheehan (1996) demonstrates the increasing costs associated with a college education, and Adams (1996) asserts that payment to student-athletes could potentially reduce the number of illegal payments taken by students. The arguments against allotting stipends to student athletes include the scholarship is sufficient payment (Dooley, 1995), athletic departments do not generate enough income to support such a program (Thompson, 1995), Title IX and other legislation would require that all students were paid regardless of sport affiliation (Rushin, 1997), and additional compensation may put the non-profit status of the NCAA in Jeopardy (Byers, 1995).

The issue of amateur status continues to be one of the most debated issues surrounding intercollegiate athletics today and compensation for student athletes is an integral facet of the conversation. Much like the rest of society, athletic directors seem to be on opposite sides of the debate as well. Branch and Crow, (1994) indicated that athletic directors felt that stipends would never occur and the desirability is highly undesirable; whereas, Drain and Ashley, (2000) posit a 21-40% likelihood that stipends will occur and this is only undesirable. Goss et. al (2004) puts forward that stipends are highly likely to occur and that they are still undesirable due to current financial hardships of most athletic departments. As time has progressed from one study to the next, research indicates a lesser chance that student athletes will have agent representation (Branch and Crow, 1994; Drain and Ashley, 2000; Goss et. al, 2004), and Goss et. al (2004) found that most athletic directors feel that legislation will be passed preventing agent representation.

Gender Equity. When dealing with Title IX compliance athletic departments appear to have three resolutions, cut men's teams, reduce men's roster sizes while increasing women's roster sizes, or increase the participation and funding of women sports. Krupa and Dunnavant (1989) predicted that men's non revenue sports would be dropped rather than the other two options, and Anderson (1999) asserts that this is in fact the case by noting the 200 male sports teams that were dropped between 1992 and 1997. However, when looking at the numbers, female participation did increase from 38,000 to 60,000 during that same time period. In terms of gender equity it appears that the solution to the issue has evolved over the past 10 years. Branch and Crow (1994), found that athletic directors not only did not think that equal funding would occur between men and women sports, but were neutral on the desirability of equality occurring. Similarly, Drain and Ashley (2000) found that athletic directors were neutral on the desirability of equal funding for male and female sports, but said that there was a possibility of it occurring. Finally, athletic directors in the Goss et. al (2004) study said that it was likely that equal funding would occur, and that a mandated increase in women's sports would occur, with a potential reduction in male sports.

NCAA. The National Collegiate Athletic Association (NCAA) is the governing body for intercollegiate athletics. The NCAA was originally created in 1906 when President Theodore Roosevelt summoned college athletic leaders to deal with the issue of safety for college football. Since then it has become the governing body of Division I, II and III level sports and organizes championships for all the recognized sports with the exception of Division I-A football. Some have argued that the NCAA has been facing the same problems for the entire duration of its existence and though research has predicted and offered solutions, most of which have been ignored (Pastore and Schneider, 2004).

Branch and Crow (1994) found that athletic directors believed that the rules needed to be revised to make them simpler and easier to follow. These findings are in conjunction with the idea that athletic directors felt that there should be stronger punishments for lack of compliance (Branch and Crow, 1994). This is supported by Drain and Ashley (2000); however; athletic directors in this study felt that individual institutions will have a stronger voice in policy matters. Athletic directors seem to have a negative perception of the future of the NCAA in general, by saying that differences between Divisions will become more blurred and the lack of efficiency will cause a splintering of the organizations (Drain and Ashley, 2000). This finding was contradicted by Goss et. al (2004) in that the majority of respondents felt that the demise of the NCAA would not happen. There was reduced hope that the rules would be simplified and that institutions would have a stronger voice in policy making (Goss et. al, 2004). Findings support that the NCAA will govern against performance enhancing drugs and the influence of professional sports over the student athlete (Drain and Ashley, 2000, Goss et. al, 2005) to major issues being face by intercollegiate athletics today.

Financial Conditions. One of the implications of Title IX is that universities need more creative ways two increase their revenue streams in order to support the numerous athletic teams that they field (Lee, 2001). Institutions that compete at the Division II level in football have an average loss of $1.2 million a year (Suggs, 2001). Even in the level of Division I, conferences and teams are growing stronger and richer while others are falling further behind thus potentially creating an environment in which 60 schools dominate intercollegiate athletics (Lee, 2001). Research has indicated a need for increased diversification of fund raising activities and point to corporate sponsorship as an area in which this diversification could be directed (Gray, 1996). Given the uniqueness of its football classics, HBCUs have an opportunity to tap into a new market that will specifically to benefit the participants of the event or even the conferences the participants are affiliated with (Goss et. al, 2004).

Drain and Ashley (2000) posited that intercollegiate athletics will begin to employ more diversified revenue streams within the next few years and this is highly desirable to athletic directors. Athletic directors felt that major capital projects to build new stadiums/ or renovate old ones will be completed to increase the sponsorship and hospitality abilities of the major revenue sports (Drain and Ashley, 2000). Corporate sponsorship will be a major impetus of the diversification of intercollegiate athletics fund raising and the government may play a role in the policy making of corporate sponsorships (e.g. alcohol and tobacco) (Drain and Ashley, 2000). Similarly, Goss et. al (2004) shows that there is an increased need for HBCUs to engage in corporate sponsorship as a method fund raising and suggest such venues as the classics as a good opportunity of them to begin.

Given the past research, the present study aimed to determine what issues and concerns existed at Division II athletic department, the desirability of the occurrence of the issues/trends, and the potential impact that the event will have on intercollegiate athletics. Secondly, given the uniqueness of HBCUs, this study sought to identify the potential differences within the Division between HBCUs and PWCUs.

METHODOLOGY

Similar to past research, this study utilized a modified Delphi technique to forecast the different trends and issues that may occur, when the event would occur, the desirability of the event, and the impact that the event will have on intercollegiate athletics. The population of the research was Division II athletic directors and senior women administrators. Senior women administrators were not a part of previous forecasting research; however, they potentially can bring some important insights into intercollegiate athletics.

In order to ascertain different trends and issues that athletic departments would face an initial fact gathering session was used. Using a web based design, an initial e-mail was sent to 30 athletic directors of HBCUs, 30 athletic directors of predominately white universities, and 30 random selected senior women administrators with a link to an online questionnaire. The questionnaire asked the respondents to list ten issues or trends that would occur in intercollegiate athletics within the next ten years. After two weeks, a follow-up e-mail was sent, thanking those who participated and asking those that have yet to participate, to do so. Ultimately, a total of 15 responses (7 AD's and 8 SWA's) were returned, which constituted of a 17% response rate. The low response rate could be attributed to the open ended form of questions, and the time of year that the survey was sent (i.e. summer). A content analysis was used as responses were written on note cards and categorized into similar responses. Similar to the Drain and Ashley (2000) study, a response was considered a "critical issue" and included in the second questionnaire if it was mentioned at least four times. Seventeen items met these criteria and were included in the second survey.

Once the initial fact gathering stage was completed a consensus building round was utilized to determine the occurrence, desirability, and the impact of the issues/trends. Given the low response of the first survey, we decided to expand the sample size for this round of data collection. Included in the sample were 30 athletics directors of PWCUs and HBCUs, and 30 senior woman administrators of PWCUs and 24 of HBCUs (6 had either no contact information or position available). An e-mail was sent to each of the respondents with a link to a second questionnaire. Four e-mails were returned reducing the sample size to 110. A total of 28 responses were collected (13 AD, 15 SWA), after two rounds of data collection.

The survey asked the respondents to determine within a timeline when the event would occur, the level of desirability of the event, and the impact that the event would have on intercollegiate athletics. A Likert type scale was utilized for the desirability of the event (1 = Very Desirable – 7 = Very Undesirable), and Impact (1 = Very Positive – 7 = Very Negative) the event might have on Division II athletics.

Data Analysis

Results were analyzed using descriptive statistics. Frequencies of PWCUs and HBCUs were utilized to create some descriptive evidence of differences between the two types of institutions. Though previous studies are very similar in nature to previous work in this area, this study differentiates greatly from the previous researchers' methodologies. Therefore, the results of the previous research will not be validated, nor will comparisons between this research and past research be addressed.

RESULTS

Timeline of Occurrence

The results indicated that there were a few trends that the majority of the respondents indicate are occurring presently in intercollegiate athletics at the Division II level. A complete evaluation of the items is listed in Table 1 and following are some of the items that were of interest. These items are: increased accountability of athletic departments to the universities that support them (present, n = 20 [71.4%]), athletics will be used as a tool to meet specific enrollment needs (present, n = 18 [64.3%]), there will be more involvement of the athletic department in the mission of the university (present, n = 14 [51.9%]), and student retention/graduation rates will become a part of the evaluation of coaches (present, n = 14 [50%]). Two of these items (increased accountability of athletic departments, and involvement of athletic departments in the university mission) are the only items that the respondents indicated would definitely occur in that none of the respondents indicated that either would never happen.

Conversely, there are a few items that the respondents indicated would never occur. These items were: Athletic scholarships will include a stipend (never, n = 15 [53.6%]), and the NCAA will make their rules easier to abide by (never n = 10 [35.7%]). One interesting note in the timeline of events is that two of the respondents indicated that stipends were already included in the athletic scholarship (present n = 2 [7.1%]). A consensus of the respondents was not found on any of the issues or trends that the respondents felt would never occur.

Desirability

The second part of the instrument asked respondents to indicate the desirability of the event occurring, and a complete comparison of the 17 issues/trends is listed in Table 2.

Table 1. Occurrence

Issue/Trend	Present						2007 - 2010						2011 - 2015						Later						Never			
	Total		PWCU		HBCU		Total		PWCU		HBCU		Total		PWCU		HBCU		Total		PWCU		HBCU		PWCU		HBCU	
	n	%	n	%	n	%	n	%	n	%	n	%	n	%	n	%	n	%	n	%	n	%	n	%	n	%	n	%
There will be increased accountability of athletic departments to the universities that support them.	20	71,4	16	72,7	4	66,7	6	21,4	5	22,7	1	16,7	1	3,6	1	4,5	0	0,0	0	0,0	0	0,0	1	16,7	0	0,0	0	0,0
Athletics will be used as a tool to meet specific enrollment needs.	18	64,3	16	72,7	2	33,3	3	10,7	2	9,1	1	14,3	1	3,6	1	4,5	0	0,0	3	10,7	1	4,5	2	33,3	2	9,1	1	16,7
There will be more involvement of athletic departments in the mission of the university.	14	51,9	12	54,5	2	40,0	8	29,6	6	27,3	2	40,0	4	14,8	3	13,6	1	20,0	1	3,6	1	4,5	0	0,0	0	0,0	0	0,0
Student retention/graduation rates will become a part of the evaluation of coaches.	14	50,0	12	54,5	2	33,3	4	14,3	1	4,5	3	42,9	4	14,3	4	18,2	0	0,0	3	10,7	3	13,6	0	0,0	2	9,1	1	16,7
Attracting and retaining Female administrators/coaches will become a priority.	13	48,1	10	45,5	3	60,0	5	18,5	3	13,6	2	28,6	5	18,5	5	22,7	0	0,0	2	7,4	2	9,1	0	0,0	2	9,1	0	0,0
More institutions will put a greater focus on sportsmanship and ethical behavior.	13	46,4	12	54,5	1	16,7	8	28,6	6	27,3	2	25,0	1	3,6	0	0,0	1	16,7	2	7,1	1	4,5	1	16,7	3	13,6	1	16,7
Academic standards to be admitted and to remain eligible to participate will be strengthened.	11	39,3	7	31,8	4	66,7	9	32,1	8	36,4	1	11,1	3	10,7	3	13,6	0	0,0	2	7,1	1	4,5	1	16,7	3	13,6	0	0,0
Graduate rates/student retention will change the type of student athlete being recruited.	10	35,7	8	36,4	2	33,3	7	25	6	27,3	1	12,5	3	10,7	3	13,6	0	0,0	4	14,3	2	9,1	2	33,3	3	13,6	1	16,7
Corporate Sponsorships will become a major source of revenue for Division II athletic departments.	8	28,6	7	31,8	1	16,7	3	10,7	3	13,6	0	0,0	6	21,4	4	18,2	2	33,3	6	21,4	3	13,6	3	50,0	5	22,7	0	0,0
Increasing tuition costs/grants-in-aid will cause a downsizing of athletic programs.	7	25,0	4	18,2	3	50,0	5	17,9	5	22,7	0	0,0	5	17,9	4	18,2	1	16,7	7	25	5	22,7	2	33,3	4	18,2	0	0,0
Women's sports will reach parity with men's sports in terms of funding.	7	25,0	7	31,8	0	0,0	4	14,3	3	13,6	1	12,5	3	10,7	2	9,1	1	16,7	6	21,4	5	22,7	1	16,7	5	22,7	3	50,0
NCAA will revise their rules to make them easier to abide by.	6	21,4	6	27,3	0	0,0	7	25	5	22,7	2	20,0	4	14,3	3	13,6	1	16,7	1	3,6	1	4,5	0	0,0	7	31,8	3	50,0
NCAA will alter the way it monitors and defines ameturism in Division II athletics.	6	21,4	6	27,3	0	0,0	11	39,3	9	40,9	2	22,2	3	10,7	1	4,5	2	33,3	3	10,7	2	9,1	1	16,7	4	18,2	1	16,7

Table 1. (Continued)

Statement	n	%	n	%	n	%	n	%	n	%	n	%	n	%	n	%	n	%	n	%	n	%	n	%	n	%	n	%	n	%
Sanctions will become more severe for breaking the rules of the NCAA.	5	17,9	2	9,1	3	50,0	11	39,3	9	40,9	2	18,2	3	10,7	2	9,1	1	16,7	4	14,3	4	18,2	0	0,0	5	17,9	5	22,7	0	0,0
Women coaches/administrators salary will be equal to their male counterparts.	5	17,9	5	22,7	0	0,0	5	17,9	5	22,7	0	0,0	3	10,7	3	13,6	0	0,0	7	25	4	18,2	3	50,0	8	28,6	5	22,7	3	50,0
Athletic scholarhsips for student athletes will include a stipend.	2	7,1	1	4,5	1	16,7	2	7,1	1	4,5	1	5,3	0	0	0	0,0	0	0,0	9	32,1	6	27,3	3	50,0	15	53,6	14	63,6	1	16,7
There will be a reduction of competitions and an emphasis on student-athlete participation in class	2	7,1	1	4,5	1	16,7	6	21,4	5	22,7	1	9,1	4	14,3	4	18,2	0	0,0	7	25	5	22,7	2	33,3	9	32,1	7	31,8	2	33,3

Table 2. Desirability

Issue/Trend	Desirable						Neutral						Undesirable					
	Total		PWCU		HBCU		Total		PWCU		HBCU		Total		PWCU		HBCU	
	n	%	n	%	n	%	n	%	n	%	n	%	n	%	n	%	n	%
More institutions will put a greater focus on sportsmanship and ethical behavior.	27	96,4	22	100	5	83,3	1	3,6	0	0,0	1	16,7	0	0	0	0,0	0	0,0
There will be more involvment of athletic departments in the mission of the university.	25	92,6	20	90,9	5	100	2	7,4	2	9,1	0	0,0	0	0	0	0,0	0	0,0
Women coaches/administrators salary will be equal to their male counterparts.	22	81,5	18	85,7	4	66,7	4	14,8	3	14,3	1	16,7	1	3,7	0	0,0	1	16,7
Attracting and retaining Female administrators/coaches will become a priority.	21	80,8	17	81,0	4	80,0	4	15,4	3	14,3	1	20,0	1	3,8	1	4,8	0	0,0
There will be increased accountability of athletic departments to the universities that support them	22	78,6	16	72,7	6	100	6	21,4	6	27,3	0	0,0	0	0	0	0,0	0	0,0
Student retention/graduation rates will become a part of the evaluation of coaches.	22	78,6	16	72,7	6	100	2	7,1	2	9,1	0	0,0	4	14,3	4	18,2	0	0,0
Women's sports will reach parity with men's sports in terms of funding.	22	78,6	17	77,3	5	83,3	6	21,4	5	22,7	1	16,7	0	0	0	0,0	0	0,0
Corporate Sponsorships will become a major source of revenue for Division II athletic departments.	21	75,0	16	72,7	5	83,3	6	21,4	5	22,7	1	16,7	1	3,6	1	4,5	0	0,0

Table 2. Desirability (Continued)

Issue/Trend	Desirable Total n	%	PWCU n	%	HBCU n	%	Neutral Total n	%	PWCU n	%	HBCU n	%	Undesirable Total n	%	PWCU n	%	HBCU n	%
NCAA will revise their rules to make them easier to abide by	21	75,0	18	81,8	3	50,0	4	14,3	1	4,5	3	50,0	3	10,7	3	13,6	0	0,0
Sanctions will become more severe for breaking the rules of the NCAA	21	75,0	18	81,8	3	50,0	5	17,9	2	9,1	3	50,0	2	7,1	2	9,1	0	0,0
Academic standards to be admitted and to remain eligible to particpate will be strengthened.	21	75,0	15	68,2	6	100	6	21,4	6	27,3	0	0,0	1	3,6	1	4,5	0	0,0
Graduate rates/student retention will change the type of student athlete being recruited.	20	74,1	16	76,2	4	66,7	5	18,5	4	19,0	1	16,7	2	7,4	1	4,8	1	16,7
NCAA will alter the way it monitors and defines ameteurism in Division II athletics.	19	67,9	17	77,3	2	33,3	9	32,1	4	18,2	3	50,0	2	7,1	1	4,5	1	16,7
Athletics will be used as a tool to meet specific enrollment needs.	16	57,1	10	45,5	6	100	7	25	7	31,8	0	0,0	5	17,9	5	22,7	0	0,0
There will be a reduction of competitions and an emphasis on student-athlete participation in class.	13	37,0	11	50,0	2	40,0	9	33,3	6	27,3	2	40,0	8	29,6	5	22,7	1	20,0
Athletic involvement for student athletes will include a stipend.	6	21,4	1	4,5	5	83,3	6	21,4	5	22,7	1	16,7	16	57,1	16	72,7	0	0,0
Increasing tuition costs/grants-in-aid will cause a downsizing of athletic programs.	4	14,3	3	13,6	1	16,7	5	17,9	4	18,2	1	16,7	19	67,9	15	68,2	4	66,7

For a better representation if the respondent indicated that the event was slight or very desirable, this was viewed as a desirable event, and conversely, the same for slightly and very undesirable. The results indicated that four of the items were either desirable or neutral, and had no undesirable responses. The items are: more institutional focus on sportsmanship and ethical behavior (desirable, n = 27 [96.4%]; neutral, n = 1 [3.6%]), there will be more involvement of the athletic department in the mission of the university (desirable, n = 25 [92.6%]; neutral, n = 2 [7.4%]), there will be increased accountability of athletic departments to the universities that support them (desirable, n = 22 [78.6%]; neutral n = 6 [21.4%]), and women's sports will reach parity with men's sports in terms of funding (desirable, n = 22 [78.6%]; neutral, n = 6 [21.4%]). Two other items demonstrated a high portion of the respondents considering the item a desirable event (women coaches/administrators salary will be equal to their male counterparts (desirable, n = 22 [81.5%]; neutral, n = 2 [7.4%]; undesirable, n = 1 [3.7%]), and attracting and retaining female administrators/coaches will become a priority (desirable, n = 21 [80.8%]; neutral, n = 4 [15.4%]; undesirable, n = 1 [3.8%]).

As far as items that were indicated as undesirable, none of the events were indicated by the respondents as being completely undesirable or neutral. However, two items denoted that they are undesirable by the majority. These items are as follows: athletic scholarships will include a stipend (desirable, n = 6 [21.4%]; neutral, n = 6 [21.4%]; undesirable, n = 16 [57.1%]), and increasing tuition costs/grants-in-aid will cause a downsizing of athletic programs (desirable, n = 4 [14.3%]; neutral n = 5 [17.9%]; undesirable, n = 19 [67.9%]).

Predicted Impact of the Event

The final section of the survey asked the respondents to signify the impact the issue/trend will have on intercollegiate athletics, and a complete listing of the comparisons is in Table 3. Similar to the results of the desirability section of the survey the responses were considered to have a positive impact in the respondents indicated either very or slight positive impact, and conversely, with a negative impact. The results show that three items reached a consensus of having either a neutral or positive impact (Attracting female coaches/administrators will become a priority (positive impact, n= 22 [81.5%]; neutral n = 5 [18.5%]), women's sports will reach a parity with men's sports in terms of funding (positive impact, n = 22 [78.6%]; neutral, n = 6 [21.4%]), and academic standards to be admitted and to remain eligible will be strengthened (positive impact, n = 21 [75%]; neutral, n = 7 [25%]). Three additional items demonstrated a strong proclivity to a positive impact occurring, and they are as follows: More institutions will put a greater focus on sportsmanship and ethical behavior (positive impact, n = 26 [92.6%]; neutral, n = 1 [3.6 %]; negative impact, n = 1 [3.6%]), there will be more involvement of athletic departments in the mission of the university (positive impact, n = 23 [85.2%]; neutral, n = 3 [11.1 %]; negative impact, n = 1 [3.7%]), and women coaches/administrators salary will be equal to their male counterparts (positive impact, n = 22 [81.5%]; neutral, n = 4 [14.8 %]; negative impact, n = 1 [3.7%]).

None of the issues/trends were indicated as having either neutral or negative impact; however, two items were felt by the majority of the respondents of having a negative impact (Increasing tuition costs/grants-in-aid will cause a downsizing of athletic programs (positive impact, n = 3 [10.7%]; neutral, n = 7 [25 %]; negative impact, n = 18 [64.3%]) and athletic scholarships will include a stipend (positive impact, n = 7 [25%]; neutral, n = 7, [25%]; negative impact, n = 14 [50%]).

Comparison of PWCUs and HBCUs

The final purpose of this study was to determine if there were any differences between the future predictions of PWCUs and HBCUs. The small sample size did not allow for any statistically significant differences; however, anecdotal evidence does appear when looking at the frequency levels of the different institution types. When comparing the results of PWCUs to HBCUs a few items are worthy of note, but none more so than the desirability and the impact of stipends for student athletes. Results indicate that 5 of the 6 respondents from an HBCU indicated that stipends were desirable and would have a positive impact; whereas, 1 of the 22 respondents from a PWCU denoted that the stipends are desirable and 2 of the 22 specified that stipends would have a positive impact. When comparing the results of PWCUs to HBCUs a few items are worthy of note, but none more so than the desirability and the impact of stipends for student athletes. Results indicate that 5 of the 6 respondents from an HBCU indicated that stipends were desirable and would have a positive impact; whereas, 1 of the 22 respondents from a PWCU denoted that the stipends are desirable and 2 of the 22 specified that stipends would have a positive impact.

Table 3. Impact

Issue/Trend	Positive Impact						No Impact						Negative Impact					
	Total		PWCU		HBCU		Total		PWCU		HBCU		Total		PWCU		HBCU	
	n	%	n	%	n	%	n	%	n	%	n	%	n	%	n	%	n	%
More institutions will put a greater focus on sportsmanship and ethical behavior.	26	92,6	21	95,5	5	83,3	1	3,6	0	0,0	1	16,7	1	3,6	1	4,5	0	0,0
There will be more involvement of athletic departments in the mission of the university.	23	85,2	20	90,9	3	60,0	3	11,1	2	9,1	1	20,0	1	3,7	0	0,0	1	20,0
Attracting and retaining Female administrators/coaches will become a priority.	22	81,5	18	81,8	4	80,0	5	18,5	4	18,2	1	20,0	0	0	0	0,0	0	0,0
Women coaches/administrators salary will be equal to their male counterparts.	22	81,5	18	85,7	4	66,7	4	14,8	3	14,3	1	16,7	1	3,7	0	0,0	1	16,7
Sanctions will become more severe for breaking the rules of the NCAA	22	78,6	19	86,4	3	50,0	4	14,3	2	9,1	2	33,3	2	7,1	1	4,5	1	16,7
Student retention/graduation rates will become a part of the evaluation of coaches.	22	78,6	17	77,3	6	100	2	7,1	1	4,5	0	0,0	4	14,3	4	18,2	0	0,0

Table 3. Impact (Continued)

Issue/Trend	Positive Impact						No Impact						Negative Impact					
	Total		PWCU		HBCU		Total		PWCU		HBCU		Total		PWCU		HBCU	
	n	%	n	%	n	%	n	%	n	%	n	%	n	%	n	%	n	%
Women's sports will reach parity with men's sports in terms of funding.	22	78,6	17	77,3	5	100	6	21,4	5	22,7	0	0,0	0	0	0	0,0	0	0,0
Corporate Sponsorships will become a major source of revenue for Division II athletic departments.	19	76,0	15	75,0	4	80,0	5	20	4	20,0	1	20,0	1	4	1	5,0	0	0,0
There will be increased accountability of athletic departments to the universities that support them	21	75,0	15	68,2	6	100	4	14,3	4	18,2	0	0,0	3	10,7	3	13,6	0	0,0
Academic standards to be admitted and to remain eligible to participate will be strengthened.	21	75,0	15	68,2	6	100	7	25	7	31,8	0	0,0	0	0	0	0,0	0	0,0
Graduate rates/student retention will change the type of student athlete being recruited.	21	75,0	17	77,3	4	66,7	6	21,4	5	22,7	1	16,7	1	3,6	0	0,0	1	16,7

Table 3. Impact (Continued)

Issue/Trend	Positive Impact						No Impact						Negative Impact					
	Total		PWCU		HBCU		Total		PWCU		HBCU		Total		PWCU		HBCU	
	n	%	n	%	n	%	n	%	n	%	n	%	n	%	n	%	n	%
NCAA will alter the way it monitors and defines ameteurism in Division II athletics.	17	60,7	15	68,2	2	33,3	9	32,1	6	27,3	3	50,0	2	7,1	1	4,5	1	16,7
NCAA will revise their rules to make them easier to abide by	16	57,1	14	63,6	2	33,3	7	25	4	18,2	3	50,0	5	17,9	4	18,2	1	16,7
Athletics will be used as a tool to meet specific enrollment needs.	16	57,1	10	45,5	6	100	7	25	7	31,8	0	0,0	5	17,9	5	22,7	0	0,0
There will be a reduction of competitions and an emphasis on student-athlete participation in class.	10	37,0	8	38,1	2	33,3	9	33,3	6	28,6	3	50,0	8	29,6	7	33,3	1	16,7
Athletic scholarhsips for student athletes will include a stipend.	7	25,0	2	9,1	5	83,3	7	25	6	27,3	1	16,7	14	50	14	63,6	0	0,0
Increasing tuition costs/grants-in-aid will cause a downsizing of athletic programs.	3	10,7	2	9,1	1	16,7	7	25	4	18,2	3	50,0	18	64,3	16	72,7	2	33,3

Corporate sponsorships will become a major source of revenue for Division II athletic departments, women's sports will reach parity with men's sports in terms of funding, and women coaches/administrators salary will be equal to their male counterparts are the three items indicated by the frequency measures (Table 1) in which there is a difference in the expectation of the occurrence. Further analysis shows that for each of these items athletic directors and senior women administrators of HBCUs feel that these events are either going to occur later than that of the PWCU counterparts, or never at all. In terms of desirability (Table 2) HBCUs reached a consensus on student retention/graduation rates will become a part of the evaluation of coaches (HBCU desirable, n = 6; PWCU desirable, n = 16, neutral, n = 2, undesirable, n = 4), Academic standards will be strengthened (HBCU desirable, n = 6; PWCU desirable, n = 15, neutral, n = 6, undesirable, n = 1), and athletics will be used as a tool to meet specific enrollment needs (HBCU desirable, n = 6; PWCU desirable, n = 10, neutral, n = 7, undesirable, n = 5). In terms of impact (Table 3), each of the items that HBCU athletic directors and senior women administrators reached consensus were felt as having a positive impact on intercollegiate athletics; whereas, the counterparts at PWCUs did not reach the same agreement. These items are as follows: athletics will be used as a tool to meet specific enrollment needs (positive, n = 10, neutral, n = 7, negative, n = 5), student retention/graduation rates will become a part of the evaluation of coaches (positive, n = 17, neutral, n = 1, negative, n = 4), and there will be increased accountability of athletic departments to the universities that support them (positive, n = 15, neutral, n = 4, negative, n = 3).

DISCUSSION

This study attempted to ascertain some of the issues and trends that will be faced by intercollegiate athletic departments competing at the Division II level. The results indicated that a majority of the items listed will have a positive impact for intercollegiate athletics (15 of the 17 items had a majority of the issues/trends as having a positive impact), and that most of the items were desirable to occur by the majority (15 of the 17 items). This could be that the athletic directors and senior women administrators that responded to the original survey listed issues or trends that they would like to occur in the next decade rather than events or issues that they may not wish to face. As represented by the data, most of the items are likely to occur in the next 10 years, with the exception of maybe stipends for student athletes.

The difference in regards to stipends by PWCUs and HBCUs is an intriguing byproduct of this research study. The research supports that HBCUs feel that student athletes should get a stipend and that this event would be beneficial to intercollegiate athletics. Though no information from this research study identifies reasons for this difference, it could be attributed to the make-up of the student body. HBCU students tend to come from less affluent areas and most work, use student loans, or federal grants to pay for their schooling. This coupled with being an athlete may leave the student in a position in which they cannot afford the day to day items necessary to survive (i.e. food, text books, etc.) Further research should be completed to determine why there is such a dichotomy between HBCUs and PWCUs in regards to stipends.

Further research should be conducted to increase the sample size of each of these issues to determine if there is a statistical difference between HBCUs and PWCUs, and if one occurs what are the causes of the dichotomy. Another area that would be interesting to study would be the predictions of coaches at the collegiate level. Coaches face many challenges in the day-to day operations of running a college level team including recruiting, ethics, NCAA compliance, scheduling competitions, etc. and these areas would be interested to further divulge. Lastly, both senior women administrators and athletic directors indicated that each of the gender related issues were desirable and would have a positive impact on intercollegiate athletics; however, this is not the case in practice and some may argue that it is getting worse. Research should be conducted to determine why there is a disconnect between what athletic directors and senior women administrators would like to occur and what is actually occurring.

This study had several limitations. The first limitation is that the sample size is too small to indicate significant differences between HBCUs and PWCUs and should be addressed by increasing the sample size in order to determine statistically significant differences. Secondly, because the survey was internet based, only those with an active e-mail account could be represented in the study, thus excluded a small portion of the entire population from being able to participate in the study. This can be corrected by using different forms of data collection similar to that of past prediction research, in which utilized mail based questionnaires. Though some of the results are consistent with past research this study is a look at the issues and trends at one specific time, and a longevity study should be completed to determine the future predictions and the methods of dealing with the issues and trends.

REFERENCES

Adams, J. (1996). Paying Athletes. *The NCAA News,* 4.

APR Statistics, (2006). www.ncaa.org. Retrieved June 1, 2006, from www.ncaa. org.

Agathe D.E., and Billings, R.B., (2000). The role of football profits in meeting Title IX gender equity regulations and policy. *Journal of Sport Management,* 14, 28-40.

Anderson, D. (1999) Men's losses in collegiate athletics. Retrieved June, 3 2006 from http://www.themat.com/etc/title9/080899.asp.

Branch, D. and Crow, R.B. (1994). Intercollegiate athletics: back to the future? *Sport marketing quarterly,* 3, 13-21.

Brown, M.C., and Davis, J.E. (2001). The historically black college as social contract, social capital, and social equalizer. *Peabody Journal of Education,* 76(1), 31-49.

Byers, W. (1995). *Unsportsmanlike conduct.* Ann Arbor: University of Michigan.

Bynum, M. (2004). After enduring decades in relative obscurity, athletic programs at historically black colleges and universities are securing their place at the sponsorship table. *Athletic Business, 71-80.*

Copeland B.W., and Kirsch, S. (1995). Perceived occupation stress among division I, II, and III athletic directors. *Journal of Sport Management,* 9, 70-77.

Dooley, V. (1995). Student-athletes well compensated. *The NCAA News,* 4-5.

Drain, T.S., and Ashley, F.B. (2000). Intercollegiate athletics: back to the future II: a comparison with Branch and Crow five years later. *Sport Marketing Quarterly,* 9, 77-84.

Fulks, (2001). Revenues and expenses of division I and II intercollegiate athletics programs. Indianapolis: The National Collegiate Athletic Association, 40-47.

Geist, A. and Pastore, D. (2002). Leadership in Division II athletic directors. *Athletics Administration,* 10-13.

Goss, B.D., Crow, R.B, Ashley, F.B., and Jubenville, C.B (2004). Qualitative trends in intercollegiate athletics at historically black colleges and universities: the impact of the NCAA structure. *International Journal of Sport Management,* 5, 367-388.

Gray, D.P. (1996). Sponsorship on campus. *Sports Marketing Quarterly,* 5(2), 29-34.

Jackson, E.N., Lyons, R., and Gooden, S.C. (2001) The marketing of black college sports. *Sport Marketing Quarterly,* 10, 138-146.

Krupa, G. and Dunnavant, K. (1989). The struggle with the downside. *Sports Inc.,* 2 (1), 33-34, 37-38.

Lee, J. (2001). Bottom-line challenges top the demands on today's Ads. *Sports Business Journal, 3(41), 31.*

Leonard, W.M. (1986). The sports experience of black college athlete: exploitation of the academy. *Int. Rev. for Soc. Of Sport, 35-48.*

Nance, R. (1996). A prescription for survival. *Sports View, 20-25.*

NCAA News, (2006). www.ncaa.org. Retrieved May, 23 2006, from www.ncaa.org.

Pastore, D. and Schneider, R., (2004). Past and future predictions of NCAA Division I intercollegiate athletics. *International Journal of Sports Management,* 5, 183-196.

Pickle, D. (2005). Willingness to cover production costs for selected event may pay off in several ways. *NCAA News Online.*

Rushin, S. (1997). Inside the moat. *Sports Illustrated,* 68.

Sage, G.H. (1998). Power and ideology of college student-athletes: student-athletes' and administrators' perceptions. *International Sports Journal,* 4, 44-55.

Schneider, R.G. (2000). Factors influencing student-athletes' perceptions of the payment of intercollegiate athletics. *International Journal of Sport Management,* 1, 296-307.

Sheehan, R.G. (1996). Keeping Score. South Bend, IN: Diamond Communications.

Sports (2006). www.ncaa.org. Retrieved May 31, 2006, from www.ncaa.org.

Suggs, W. (2000). Gap grows between the haves and the have nots in college sports. *The chronicle of higher education,* A73.

Suggs, W. (2001). Can anyone do anything about college sports? *The Chronicle of Higher Education,* A50.

Thompson, G. (1995). Pay for play. *Black issues in higher education,* 3.

In: Sports and Athletics Developments
Editor: James H. Humphrey, pp. 81-100

ISBN: 978-1-60456-205-7
© 2008 Nova Science Publishers, Inc.

Chapter 5

COACH AND ATHLETE BURNOUT: THE ROLE OF COACHES' DECISION-MAKING STYLE

Brandonn S. Harris and Andrew C. Ostrow
West Virginia University

ABSTRACT

Recent burnout research has examined coaches and athletes collectively to determine the influence of coach behaviors on coach and athlete burnout. Results revealed a potential incongruity between decision-making behaviors and their influence on coach and athlete burnout. Therefore, the present study examined relationships between decision-making styles of coaches and burnout among coaches and athletes; gender influence on burnout was also examined. Collegiate swimmers and swimming coaches completed questionnaires assessing burnout and decision-making behaviors. Results revealed a significant relationship between athlete burnout and autocratic coaching behaviors. A significant inverse relationship emerged between athlete burnout and democratic behaviors. Significant main effects were found for democratic behaviors on exhaustion and depersonalization subscales; swimmers perceiving fewer democratic behaviors scored higher on these subscales. No significant relationships or gender differences were found with the coaches. Results suggest that coaches eliciting feedback from athletes could reduce the likelihood of burnout among those athletes without predisposing themselves.

Keywords: Coach and Athlete Burnout, Decision-Making, Leadership.

Burnout has become a topic of increasing interest to the sport community with some even suggesting that burnout has become synonymous with sports (Lai & Wiggins, 2003). When asked what feelings they associate with being burned out, athletes and coaches often cite internal and external sources of pressure, physical and mental exhaustion, mood changes, increased anxiety, and lack of caring (Weinberg & Gould, 2007). As both athletes and coaches experiencing burnout can end up mentally and physically withdrawing from a sport they once used to enjoy, it is apparent that a great deal of significance rests in understanding burnout.

With the coach and athlete populations having received research attention individually, recent studies have examined both groups collectively to determine the influence of coaching behaviors on coach and athlete burnout (Price & Weiss, 2000; Udry, Gould, Bridges, & Tuffey, 1997; Vealey, Armstrong, Comar, & Greenleaf, 1998). Related research on coaching behaviors has also noted that discrepancies between athletes' perceived and preferred leader/coach behaviors can contribute to dissatisfaction with athletes' sport experiences (Chelladurai, 1984). While this may be true, coach and athlete burnout may be another factor to consider that could result from this discrepancy. In noting that athletes cite severe practice conditions as the most important reason for their own burnout, Vealey et al. (1998) suggested the behaviors of coaches who are typically responsible for the practice conditions may be a critical component worthy of consideration in the occurrence of burnout among athletes. Although this premise guided their own research on athlete burnout, relatively little attention has been given to the effect coaches' behaviors, particularly decision-making styles, have on the occurrence of burnout in both coaches and athletes.

RESEARCH REGARDING DECISION-MAKING AND BURNOUT IN SPORT

One relevant study to this line of research in the coaching population was conducted by Dale and Weinberg (1989). These authors studied leadership style and burnout in coaches and found those utilizing a consideration style evidenced greater emotional exhaustion and depersonalization, two common indicators of burnout. The authors suggested coaches with this style of leadership may become more emotionally involved with their teams, often giving more to their team than themselves. Price and Weiss (2000) found similar results in their research. Their study revealed that coaches reporting greater levels of burnout were perceived by their athletes to utilize democratic decision-making behaviors regarding their sport. However, in contrast to these two studies, Kelley, Eklund, and Ritter-Taylor (1999) found a democratic style of leadership to be associated with lower levels of burnout among coaches.

This line of burnout and leadership behavior research has also yielded some potentially troubling results, specifically the potential incongruity between decision-making styles and burnout among athletes and coaches that becomes apparent when examining the athlete burnout and leadership research. Vealey et al. (1998) examined the influence of perceived coaching behaviors on athlete burnout. Results indicated that athletes who scored higher on a burnout inventory also perceived their coach's leadership style to be more autocratic in nature. Price and Weiss (2000) also found that athletes reported higher levels of burnout in response to perceived autocratic coaching behaviors and less burnout in response to a democratic style of decision-making.

Collectively, these studies suggest that a decision-making style of coaches that has been linked to higher levels of burnout in coaches (democratic) is one that may aid in protecting athletes from experiencing burnout. Further, a decision-making style of coaches that has been correlated with higher levels of burnout in athletes (autocratic) is one that might reduce the likelihood of coaches experiencing burnout.

RESEARCH REGARDING GENDER AND BURNOUT IN SPORT

In addition to leadership influences on coach and athlete burnout, research has examined the role gender plays in coach burnout; however, equivocal findings have been found (Davenport, 1998). Caccese and Mayerberg (1984) administered the Maslach Burnout Inventory (Maslach & Jackson, 1981) to 231 collegiate head coaches. Their results indicated that female coaches experienced significantly higher levels of burnout denoted by greater levels of emotional exhaustion and lower levels of personal accomplishments than their counterparts. No gender differences were found regarding the depersonalization subscale. Results have been mirrored by other studies regarding the emotional exhaustion subscale (Kelley, 1994; Kelley, et al., 1999; Pastore & Judd, 1993; Vealey, Udry, Zimmerman, & Soliday, 1992). However, Pastore and Judd (1993) and Vealey and colleagues (1992) were unable to demonstrate any gender differences regarding the personal accomplishment subscale. While many of these studies have found no gender differences regarding the depersonalization subscale of the MBI, others have suggested males experience greater levels of depersonalization than females (Dale & Weinberg, 1989). It can be concluded that gender differences in burnout among coaches needs further examination to help clarify the inconsistent findings of the previous research.

Interestingly, gender differences in burnout among athletes have received little research attention. Lai and Wiggins (2003) examined burnout perceptions in collegiate soccer players. Their hypotheses were formulated based on gender and burnout research conducted with coaches. They found that while burnout symptoms significantly increased over the course of a competitive season, no gender differences in burnout perceptions were present. The authors suggested that future research address possible gender differences in burnout among athletes so that future researchers may formulate hypotheses based on previous athlete burnout literature rather than the available coach research.

The results of the abovementioned research have left the burnout arena with several significant issues that warrant future attention. First, the relationship of decision-making style and burnout among coaches has yet to be clearly identified as research has yielded inconsistent findings. An additional issue of concern regards the incongruity between athlete and coach burnout and coaches' decision-making behaviors. Research has suggested that the decision-making style that has been linked to coach burnout (democratic or consideration) is one that may keep athletes from experiencing burnout. Further, the decision-making style linked to athlete burnout (autocratic) may be one that safeguards coaches from experiencing burnout. Additional research is needed to examine this relationship and ultimately reduce the potential of either group experiencing burnout. Further, the inconsistent results regarding gender differences in burnout among coaches and the paucity of research examining gender differences in burnout among athletes highlights the need for empirical research attention in both of these areas as well.

Therefore, the present research examined the relationship between perceived coaches' decision-making style and athletes' and coaches' burnout levels in the competitive sport of collegiate swimming. Secondary purposes included assessing gender differences in burnout within the coach and athlete populations, as well as the interaction between decision-making style and gender on burnout dimensions.

Both athlete and coach burnout was assessed utilizing the multidimensional theoretical framework established by Raedeke and Smith (2001), which defines burnout as a psychological syndrome of emotional/physical exhaustion, reduced sense of accomplishment, and sport devaluation (Raedeke, 1997; Raedeke & Smith, 2001). The multidimensional model of leadership (Chelladurai & Saleh, 1980) served as the theoretical framework for assessing coach and athlete perceptions of leadership behaviors, in particular, democratic and autocratic decision-making. A democratic decision-making style was defined as a style in which coaches permit participation by athletes in decisions regarding team goals, practice methods, and game tactics and strategies. An autocratic decision-making style was defined as a style in which a coach exercises independence in decision making and stresses their authority in dealing with their athletes (Chelladurai & Doherty, 1998; Chelladurai & Saleh, 1980).

It was hypothesized that as athletes perceive their coach's decision-making style to be more autocratic in nature, their own reported levels of burnout will increase. Further, as athletes perceive their coach's decision-making style to be democratic their own reported levels of burnout will decrease. Second, it was hypothesized that as coaches report more of autocratic style for decision-making their reported levels of burnout will decrease. Further, as coaches report more of a democratic decision-making style their reported levels of burnout will increase.

It was also hypothesized that male athletes who perceive more autocratic behaviors will report less burnout than their female counterparts. The same relationship was expected in the coaching population. It was also hypothesized that coaches who are high in autocratic behaviors and low in democratic behaviors will report less burnout than those coaches who are higher in democratic behaviors and lower in autocratic behaviors. Athletes who perceive their coaches to be higher in autocratic behaviors and lower in democratic behaviors will report more burnout than those athletes who report a perception of higher democratic and lower autocratic behaviors.

METHODS

Participants

Athlete participants included male (n=38) and female (n=53) collegiate swimmers (N=91). Seventy-six collegiate swimmers competed in NCAA Division I (n=49) and Division II (n=27) programs. An additional 15 collegiate swimmers competing outside of NCAA governance also participated in the study. Athletes' ages ranged from 19 to 25 years with a mean age of 19.98 years (SD= 2.38). The average number of years athletes reported swimming competitively was 11.43 (SD=3.23). Athletes also reported spending an average of 20.93 hours per week on swimming-related obligations (SD=4.74).

The coaching sample included thirty-six collegiate swimming coaches who were affiliated with NCAA Division I (n=13), Division II (n=8), and Division III (*n*=9) swimming programs. Five coaches did not report their divisional status and one international collegiate swimming coach was employed outside of the United States. Twenty-three of the coaches were male and eight were female. Gender was not reported by five participants. The mean age of coach participants was 39.64 years (*SD*=9.94) with ages ranging from 23 to 58 years. The average number of years coaches reported coaching competitive swimming was 18.75 (*SD*=9.77). Coaches also reported spending an average of 50.28 hours per week on coaching-related duties (*SD*=16.82).

Measures Completed by Athletes

Swimmer Demographic Information Form. All collegiate swimmers completed a demographic information form that assessed personal characteristics, number of years swimming competitively, number of hours spent per week on swimming-related duties, and variables pertaining to their academic level and level of competition.

Athlete Burnout Questionnaire (ABQ). The Athlete Burnout Questionnaire (Raedeke & Smith, 2001) was used to assess levels of burnout in swimmers. This multidimensional inventory contains 15 items that assess three subscales of sport burnout: a) reduced sense of accomplishment, b) emotional and physical exhaustion, and c) sport devaluation. Participants respond to the degree each item applies to him or her using a Likert-type scale ranging from 1 ("almost never) to 5 ("almost always"). The psychometric properties of this instrument have been deemed adequate as construct validity and test-retest reliability were established during the inventory's construction (Raedeke & Smith, 2001).

Leadership Scale for Sports (LSS: Athlete Perception). To assess athletes' perceived decision-making style of their coaches, Chelladurai and Saleh's (1978, 1980) Leadership Scale for Sports was utilized. The LSS is a 40-item inventory that assesses several dimensions of coaches' leadership behaviors: a) social support, b) training and instruction, c) positive feedback, d) autocratic behavior, and e) democratic behavior. In completing the leadership perception inventory athletes are asked to respond by indicating how often their coach exhibits particular leadership behaviors. Their answers for each question are anchored from 1 ("always") to 5 ("never").

The psychometric properties of the LSS were demonstrated during its construction and included test-retest reliability (coefficients ranged from .71 to .82) and subscale internal consistencies (Chelladurai & Saleh, 1980). Cronbach's alpha coefficients for the five subscales were above .70 except the autocratic subscale. Because previous research has also found the autocratic subscale to have questionable internal consistency (Dwyer & Fischer, 1988) this component of the LSS was of concern for the present research. To compensate for the potential inadequate reliability of this subscale, improvements to its internal consistency were made based on previous research by Price and Weiss (2000). These authors added three items to the autocratic subscale for their study which resulted in adequate reliability for this subscale. These items were also used for the present study with those authors' permission.

Measures Completed by Coaches

Swimming Coach Demographic Information Form. All collegiate swimming coaches completed a demographic information form that assessed personal characteristics, number of years coaching swimming competitively, number of hours spent per week on swimming-related duties, and variables pertaining to their academic level and level of competition.

Coach Burnout Questionnaire (CBQ). Because there is no known sport-specific coaching burnout measure available to date, a modified version of the Athlete Burnout Questionnaire was developed to assess burnout levels in coaches. The principal investigator modified each of the 15 items in the original questionnaire to reflect coaching rather than playing their respective sport. For example, "I'm accomplishing many worthwhile things in swimming" was changed to "I'm accomplishing many worthwhile things in coaching swimming." After being modified, the coach version of the inventory was submitted to an expert panel of four former competitive swimmers and coaches/teachers who reviewed the original and modified version of the questionnaire and examined fit, clarity, and meaning of the revised items. No items were found by the panel to be inappropriately modified. This modified version appeared to have content validity and served as the Coach Burnout Questionnaire.

Leadership Scale for Sports (LSS: Coach Perception). The coach perception version of the LSS was used to assess coaches' perceptions of their own decision-making behaviors. The inventory was created along with the other versions of the scale using the same procedure previously described for the collegiate swimmer sample. Previous research has demonstrated adequate psychometric properties of this version of the LSS (Turman, 2003). To combat the potentially inadequate reliability of the autocratic subscale, the same additional three items that were added to the athlete perception version were also used for the coach perception version.

Procedures

Athletes. Data from collegiate swimmers were collected at the World Swimming Championships held in the Midwest United States. Those collegiate swimmers participating in or volunteering at the Championships who were willing to participate were given a counterbalanced packet containing a cover letter and the study's inventories and asked to place the forms in the envelope provided once completed. To increase the sample size of collegiate swimmers, additional data were collected from collegiate swimmers across collegiate athletic programs in the southeast region of the United States. Those collegiate swimmers who were willing to participate were given a counterbalanced packet containing the questionnaires and asked to place the inventories in an envelope once finished. Between both rounds of data collection, 22 athletes who were competing in the Championships were sampled. Sixty-nine collegiate swimmers not participating in the event were also sampled.

Coaches. Data from collegiate swimming coaches were collected at a world swimming coach's clinic held in the Midwest. Those collegiate swimming coaches willing to participate (n=25) were given a counterbalanced packet containing a cover letter and the study's inventories and asked to place the inventories in an envelope once finished. To increase the sample size of swimming coaches, additional data were obtained by uploading the coach inventories on the Internet under the domain of the university the researcher was affiliated with. With permission from the organization's director, members of a collegiate swimming coaches' organization received an e-mail explaining the purpose and procedures of the study in addition to a request for their participation. Those who were willing to complete the inventories (n=11) followed a link to a webpage containing electronic versions of the study's instruments for completion. Previous research has evaluated the psychometric equivalency of Internet-based research and found that data collection on the web is a valid and reliable method of acquiring data similar to that obtained when using traditional paper and pencil methods (Metzger, Kristof, & Yoest, 2003; Meyerson & Tryon, 2003).

RESULTS

Preliminary Analyses for Collegiate Swimmers

To assess the reliability of the ABQ and LSS: Athlete Perception subscales, internal consistencies were calculated using Cronbach's alpha coefficients (See

Table 1). All alpha coefficients were found to be above .70. Descriptive data for swimmers' perceptions of coaches' decision-making style for those subscales of the LSS in addition to their reported levels of burnout of each subscale of the ABQ can also be found in Table 1. The means for athletes' perception of their coach's decision-making style are comparable to those reported by Chelladurai (personal communication, March 1, 2004). An analysis of those studies using the athlete perception version of the LSS yielded an average democratic score of 3.05 (SD= .71) and an average mean for the autocratic scores of 2.64 (SD=.72). Norms for the ABQ are not yet available for comparison with the present study's results.

To examine any potential differences in the data obtained from those collegiate swimmers competing in the World Swimming Championships and those swimmers who did not compete in the event, independent sample t-tests were utilized. The only significant difference between the two groups of collegiate swimmers was on the democratic subscale of the LSS (t (89) = -2.5, p<.05).

Table 1. Internal consistency and descriptive statistics for intercollegiate swimmers (N=91) and coaches (N=36)

	Cronbach α	M	SD
ATHLETES			
ABQ			
Exhaustion	.91	3.06	.890
Sport Devaluation	.80	2.15	.803
Reduced Sense of Accomplishment	.79	2.15	.702
LSS			
Perceived Autocratic Behaviors	.80	2.76	.744
Perceived Democratic Behaviors	.81	3.30	.711
COACHES			
CBQ			
Exhaustion	.94	2.73	.984
Sport Devaluation	.88	2.03	.836
Reduced Sense of Accomplishment	.81	2.07	.671
LSS			
Perceived Autocratic Behaviors	.61	2.62	.470
Perceived Democratic Behaviors	.76	3.12	.492

Those competing in the Championships reported perceiving significantly more democratic behaviors of their coaches than did those swimmers not competing in the event. It should be noted, however, that the mean difference between group scores was .38 and was not deemed practically significant for the purposes of the present study. Therefore, both athletic groups were combined into one group for the purpose of subsequent data analyses.

Relationship between Perceived Decision-Making Style and Burnout among Swimmers

To examine the relationship between collegiate swimmers' perceived decision-making style of their coaches and their own reported levels of burnout, Pearson product-moment correlations were computed (see Table 2). The results revealed a statistically significant inverse relationship between swimmers' perception of a democratic decision-making style and their reported levels of burnout on all three subscales. Correlation coefficients ranged from $r= -.28$ to $-.33$ ($p<.01$). Results also revealed significant relationships between swimmers' perception of an autocratic decision-making style of their coaches and their reported levels of burnout on all three subscales. Correlation coefficients from this analysis ranged from $r= .22$ to $.32$ ($p<.05$).

Table 2. Pearson product correlation coefficients for burnout and decision-making style among collegiate swimmers ($N=91$) and collegiate swimming coaches ($N=36$)

	Autocratic	Democratic
ATHLETES		
Exhaustion	.25*	-.28**
Sport Devaluation	.32**	-.33**
Reduced Sense of Accomplishment	.22*	-.28**
COACHES		
Exhaustion	.02	-.11
Sport Devaluation	-.11	-.02
Reduced Sense of Accomplishment	-.24	.11

*$p<.05$
**$p<.01$

Gender, Autocratic Decision-Making Style, and Burnout among Swimmers

To assess interactions between collegiate swimmers' gender and a perceived coaches' autocratic decision-making style on their burnout levels, three, two-way (gender x high/low autocratic) ANOVAs were utilized. Each burnout subscale served as a dependent variable for the ANOVAs conducted. Collegiate swimmers' scores on the perceived autocratic decision-making behavior subscale of the LSS were recoded into either high or low autocratic perception categories. A median split was used to determine if scores were categorized as high or low. Those scores above the median were classified as high autocratic perception and those below classified as low autocratic perception.

The results of the ANOVAs revealed no statistically significant interactions between gender and autocratic perceptions of collegiate swimmers on any of the three subscales of burnout. Further examination revealed no significant main effects for gender or high/low autocratic perception on any of the three burnout subscales.

Gender, Democratic Decision-Making Style, and Burnout among Swimmers

Three, two-way (gender x high/low democratic) ANOVAs were also computed to examine any interactions between collegiate swimmers' gender and a perceived coaches' democratic decision-making style on these athletes' own levels of burnout. Again, each burnout subscale was used as a dependent variable. Swimmers' scores on the perceived democratic decision-making behavior subscale of the LSS were recoded as being either a high or low democratic perception. Similar to the autocratic scale, a median split was used to determine if scores were categorized as high or low.

The results of the ANOVAs revealed no significant interactions between gender and democratic perceptions of collegiate swimmers on any of the three burnout subscales. No significant main effects were found for gender on any of the burnout subscales. However, a significant main effect was found for perceptions of democratic behaviors with regard to the exhaustion burnout subscale (F (1, 87) = 6.13, $p<.05$, $\eta^2=.07$). Those swimmers perceiving their coach to use a high degree of democratic decision-making behaviors reported significantly less emotional and physical exhaustion than those reporting their coaches to be less democratic. A significant main effect was also found for perceptions of democratic behaviors regarding the sport devaluation burnout subscale (F (1, 87) = 7.23, $p<.01$, $\eta^2= .08$). Collegiate swimmers perceiving their coach as using a high degree of democratic decision-making behaviors reported significantly less sport devaluation than those swimmers reporting their coaches to be less democratic.

The Influence of Both Decision-Making Styles on Swimmers' Burnout

Three, two-way (high/low autocratic x high/low democratic) ANOVAs were also computed to examine any interactions between both decision-making styles and burnout among collegiate swimmers. Again, each burnout subscale was used as a dependent variable. Swimmers' scores on the perceived democratic and autocratic decision-making behavior subscales of the LSS were recoded as being either a high or low perception. A median split was again used to determine if scores were categorized as high or low.

The results revealed no significant interactions between both decision-making styles on collegiate swimmers' levels of burnout. Significant main effects were found for the democratic subscales on the exhaustion (F (1, 87) = 5.73, $p<.05$, $\eta^2=$ .06) and sport devaluation (F (1, 87)= 5.52, $p<.05$, $\eta^2=.06$) burnout subscales. Collegiate swimmers perceiving their coaches to use a higher degree of democratic decision-making behaviors reported significantly less burnout on these subscales than those swimmers reporting a low perception of democratic decision-making behaviors.

Does Perception of Decision-Making Style Predict Burnout among Swimmers?

Because it was hypothesized that collegiate swimmers' perception of their coach's decision-making style would influence their own reported levels of burnout, it was logical to ascertain the predictive value of decision-making style on swimmers' burnout. To examine this, three stepwise multiple regression analyses were conducted. Each burnout subscale served as one of the criterion variables. To determine if any additional demographic predictor variables should be included in the analyses, in addition to testing for multicolinearity, a Pearson product-moment correlation matrix was utilized. The results revealed no significant relationships between athletes' demographic information (e.g. number of years swimming competitively, number of hours per week spent on swimming-related duties) and any of the three burnout subscales. Therefore, no additional demographic variables were included in the regression analyses. Neither predictor variables (autocratic decision-making style, democratic decision-making style) were found to be highly correlated with one another suggesting multicolinearity was not of concern.

The only statistically significant predictor of the emotional and physical exhaustion component of burnout was the perception of a democratic decision-making style (F (1, 89) =7.39, $p<.01$). This model was only found to account for just under 8% of the variance in the exhaustion burnout subscale ($R^2=.078$). Two models were found to account for a statistically significant amount of the variance in the sport devaluation subscale of burnout. The most parsimonious of the two found perceptions of both a democratic and autocratic decision-making style to be significant predictors of depersonalization (F (2, 89) =8.49, $p<.001$). This model, while significant, only accounted for about 16% of the variance in the criterion variable (R^2=.163). For the reduced sense of accomplishment subscale of burnout, a model containing only a perception of democratic decision-making behaviors accounted for a statistically significant amount of the variance (F (1,89) =7.25, p<.01). This model was found to account for only about 7% of the variance (R^2= .076).

Preliminary Analyses for Collegiate Swimming Coaches

To assess the reliability of the CBQ and LSS: Coach Perception subscales, internal consistencies were calculated using Cronbach's alpha coefficients (See Table 1). Reliability coefficients ranged from .80 to .93 for the three burnout subscales. Cronbach's alpha coefficients for the perceptions of democratic and autocratic decision-making behaviors were lower. This was particularly true for the autocratic subscale for which its low reliability has been reported in previous research (Dwyer & Fischer, 1988).

Descriptive data for swimming coaches' perceptions of each decision-making style in addition to their reported levels of burnout can also be found in Table 1. Coaches in the present study reported using significantly more democratic than autocratic behaviors. These results are similar to those found by Dwyer and Fischer (1988) whose sample of wrestling coaches yielded a comparable pattern.

To examine any differences between coaches surveyed via paper and pencil questionnaires at the swimming coaching clinic and those coaches completing inventories over the Internet, independent samples t-tests were utilized. The results revealed no significant mean score differences between the two groups on any of the inventories' subscales. Therefore, both groups of data were combined for subsequent analyses.

Relationship between Perceived Decision-Making Style and Burnout among Coaches

To examine the relationship between collegiate swimmers coaches' perceived decision-making style and their own reported levels of burnout, Pearson product-moment correlations were computed (see Table 2). The results revealed no statistically significant relationships between the perception of possessing an autocratic or democratic decision-making style and coaches' scores on any of the three burnout subscales.

Gender, Decision-Making Style, and Burnout among Coaches

To assess any differences in collegiate swimming coaches' gender on their burnout levels, three independent *t*-tests were utilized. Each burnout subscale served as a dependent variable. No significant differences were found between males and females on any of the burnout subscales.

To examine differences in burnout between coaches categorized as using high versus low levels of democratic or autocratic decision-making behaviors, six additional independent *t*-tests were utilized. Three *t*-test analyses were computed for each decision-making style, one for each of the three burnout subscales serving as the dependent variable. Collegiate swimming coaches' scores on their perceived autocratic and democratic decision-making behavior subscales of the LSS were recoded into either high or low perceptions. A median split was used to determine if scores were categorized as high or low. No significant differences were found on any of the three burnout subscales between those coaches classified as using a high or low degree of democratic or autocratic decision-making behaviors.

DISCUSSION

The Influence of Decision-Making Style on Collegiate Swimmers' Burnout

The primary purpose of the present research was to examine the relationship between the perceived decision-making style of coaches and burnout among coaches and athletes. The most significant finding was the link established between collegiate swimmers' perception of their coach's decision-making style and their own reported levels of burnout. As hypothesized for the athlete sample, collegiate swimmers' levels of burnout on all three subscales were significantly related to their perception of coaches' use of autocratic and democratic decision-making styles. As swimmers perceived their coach to utilize more of an autocratic decision-making style, swimmers' reported levels of burnout on all three subscales increased. Further, as swimmers perceived their coach to utilize more of a democratic decision-making style, their reported levels of burnout on all three subscales decreased.

The relationships between swimmers' perceived decision-making style of their coach and their reported level of burnout were further confirmed by the results of the two-way ANOVAs and regression analyses. Collegiate swimmers perceiving their coaches to be more democratic in their decision-making reported significantly less burnout on these subscales than those swimmers' perceiving their coaches to use fewer democratic decision-making behaviors. In addition, perception of decision-making style was found to significantly predict all three subscales of burnout among collegiate swimmers. Collectively, these results suggest that collegiate swimmers' perception of their coach's decision-making style, particularly a democratic style of decision-making, has some influence on swimmers' reported levels of burnout.

The results of the swimmers' data mirror those of previous research examining the influences of coach leadership on athlete burnout within a multidimensional model of leadership (e.g. Price & Weiss, 2000; Vealey et al., 1998). Because democratic coaches elicit feedback from their athletes regarding decisions about their team, these athletes may perceive to have more control over and meaning in their sport participation. These perceptions may help act as a buffer against the physical and psychological stressors that, over time, can eventually lead to burnout. Contrastingly, autocratic coaches do not invite feedback from their athletes. This could contribute to a lack of perceived control and meaning among athletes regarding their sport involvement and could partially contribute to an extreme training environment that Vealey et al. (1998) noted athletes cite as the most significant cause of burnout. The results also support the findings of Udry and colleagues (1997), that suggested athletes coping with burnout often view their sport interactions with important others (including coaches) as more negative than positive. The perception of an autocratic decision-making style of their coach could contribute to collegiate swimmers' negative perception of "important others."

It is of interest that swimmers' perception of a democratic decision-making style emerged from the analyses as the more salient of the two types of decision-making styles linked to burnout levels in swimmers. A likely explanation for this finding may rest in the type of sport used for the present research. Weinberg and Gould (2007) noted that athletes participating in interactive, team sports may prefer more of an autocratic style of decision-making than athletes taking part in a coactive sport such as swimming. Partially due to the nature of their sport, swimmers' responses to the inventories may have reflected the preference for a democratic style which would help explain why more democratic than autocratic behaviors were reported by both swimmers and swimming coaches.

The secondary purposes of the present research were to examine the influence of gender and decision-making style on collegiate swimmers' burnout, in addition to the interaction of both decision-making styles on swimmers' burnout. It was hypothesized that male collegiate swimmers perceiving their coach to utilize more autocratic decisions would report less burnout than females. The results of the analyses did not support this hypothesis. Further, collegiate swimmers did not significantly differ between genders on their level of burnout on any of the three subscales. Although males have been found to prefer an autocratic style of decision-making more than females (Chelladurai & Saleh, 1978; Chelladurai & Carron, 1983; Turman, 2003), it may be that this preference does little to influence the prevalence of burnout among male versus female athletes. The failure to reveal significant gender differences in burnout among athletes does, however, support previous research conducted by Lai and Wiggins (2003). In conducting their research, these authors utilized coach burnout research to formulate their hypotheses regarding gender differences. Because little research has examined gender differences in burnout among athletes, it is important that future studies do so in the hopes that such hypotheses can be made using the results of athlete data rather than that of coaches.

It was also of interest that the two decision-making styles did not interact significantly to influence burnout among collegiate swimmers. This suggests that for the collegiate swimmers and swimming coaches surveyed, a particular combination of both decision-making styles did not influence the degree of burnout either group experienced. Prior to this study, research had not examined the potential interaction between these two distinct leadership characteristics.

The Influence of Decision-Making Style on Collegiate Swimming Coaches' Burnout

Another purpose of this study was also to examine the relationship between coaches' perception of their decision-making style and coaches' reported levels of burnout. It was hypothesized that as collegiate swimming coaches perceived themselves to utilize more of a democratic style of decision-making, their reported levels of burnout would increase. Further, as these coaches reported more of an autocratic style of decision-making, their levels of burnout would decrease. The results of the analyses did not support this hypothesis; collegiate swimming coaches' perception of their decision-making style was not found to be significantly related to any of the three burnout subscales. Subsequent analyses confirmed this finding as coaches classified as being high in their use of autocratic or democratic decision-making behaviors did not significantly differ from one another on any of the three burnout subscales. There were no differences in burnout revealed between male and female coaches as well. Finally, perception of decision-making style did not significantly predict burnout in collegiate swimming coaches.

Several propositions can be offered in understanding why these results emerged. One must acknowledge the possibility that coaches responded to the questionnaires in a socially desirable manner. In fact, previous research has masked the true nature of burnout questionnaires to account for the negative connotation associated with the construct of burnout (e.g. Gould, Udry, Tuffey, & Loehr, 1996b). The lack of willingness among coaches to express their true levels of burnout and style of decision-making could have potentially contributed to the findings of the present study.

The accuracy of the coaches' responses to the study's questionnaires, particularly the LSS, may also be worthy of consideration. Research has found that coaches' perceptions of their own leadership behaviors are less accurate than those of the athletes they coach (Smoll & Smith, 1981). It is possible that a portion of coaches sampled in the present study misrepresented their decision-making behaviors on the LSS due to an inaccurate perception of those behaviors, which could influence the results of the analyses conducted on the swimming coaches' data.

The failure to reveal gender differences among coaches on any of the three burnout subscales is not surprising when one takes into consideration the equivocal findings of previous research (Davenport, 1998). Caccese and Mayerberg (1984) found that female coaches experienced significantly higher levels of burnout denoted by greater levels of emotional exhaustion and lower levels of personal accomplishments than their male counterpart. Similar results have been found in other studies regarding the emotional exhaustion subscale (Kelley, 1994; Kelley et al., 1999; Pastore & Judd, 1993; Vealey et al., 1992) with others unable to demonstrate gender differences among the personal accomplishment subscale (Pastore & Judd, 1993; Vealey et al., 1992). Where some have found no gender differences in depersonalization, other researchers have suggested males experience greater levels of depersonalization than females (Dale & Weinberg, 1989). Additional research is clearly warranted that targets the potential gender differences among both coaches and athletes.

Finally, one has to consider the reported levels of burnout by both athletes and coaches in the present study. The sample of collegiate swimmers and swimming coaches obtained were not experiencing a high degree of burnout. Further, because the ABQ and CBQ are newer instruments used in the assessment of sport burnout, norms are not available for comparison. It is possible that many of the swimmers participating in the study, particularly those swimmers competing in the Championships, were surveyed immediately following a tapering period of their training in preparation for this significant competition. Because these athletes had not recently been exposed to the extreme training conditions that swimmers typically endure, their reported levels of burnout may have been slightly lower.

IMPLICATIONS AND FUTURE DIRECTIONS

The results of the present research revealed that collegiate swimmers' perception of their coaches' decision-making style has some degree of influence on burnout levels reported by those swimmers. Thus, it could be suggested that coaches take into consideration the degree to which they elicit feedback from their athletes regarding team-related decisions. By eliciting feedback from athletes, coaches could help create a feeling of control and meaningfulness among athletes that act as a buffer against experiencing burnout. This idea is further supported by the fact that results did not show collegiate swimming coaches' decision-making style was related to or predictive of coach burnout. Coaches who utilize a democratic style of decision-making with their team might help prevent burnout among their players without enhancing their own likelihood of experiencing the same.

Future burnout research should continue to examine the relationship between coaches' leadership variables and their impact on both coach and athlete burnout. A useful approach would be to incorporate qualitative research methods in burnout investigations of coaches and athletes experiencing a high degree of burnout as has been done in the past (e.g. Gould, Tuffey, Udry, & Loehr, 1996a). This would be particularly helpful with a coach population, as little qualitative burnout research has been done with this group.

Additional research attention should also be given to the assessment of burnout within the sport domain. Because the ABQ was developed recently, norms for the subscales and additional validation of the instrument have yet to be provided. The present research provided additional support for the internal consistency of this measure, although future research should continue to validate its psychometric properties across various sport types and establish norms for each of its subscales to compare future research with. The present research also provided preliminary support for a measure to assess sport burnout in coaches. To date, no sport burnout measure is available for the coach population. The internal consistencies found with the CBQ were high and a promising indication that such a measure could be developed and validated.

REFERENCES

Caccese, T., & Mayerberg, C. (1984). Gender differences in perceived burnout of college coaches. *Journal of Sport Psychology, 6,* 279-288.

Chelladurai, P. (1984). Discrepancy between preferences and perceptions of leadership behavior and satisfaction of athletes in varying sports. *Journal of Sport Psychology, 6,* 27-41.

Chelladurai, P., & Carron, A.V. (1983). Athletic maturity and preferred leadership. *Journal of Sport Psychology, 5,* 371-380.

Chelladurai, P., & Doherty, A. (1998). Styles of decision making in coaching. In J. Williams (Ed.), *Applied sport psychology: Personal growth to peak performance* (pp.115-126). Mountain View, CA: Mayfield Publishing Company.

Chelladurai, P., & Saleh, S.D. (1978). Preferred leadership in sports. *Canadian Journal of Applied Sport Sciences, 3,* 85-92.

Chelladurai, P., & Saleh, S.D. (1980). Dimensions of leader behavior in sports: Development of a leadership scale. *Journal of Sport Psychology, 2,* 34-45.

Dale, J., & Weinberg, R. (1989). The relationship between coaches' leadership style and burnout. *The Sport Psychologist, 3,* 1-13.

Davenport, M. (1998). *A descriptive analysis of the burnout of rowing coaches over a competitive season.* Unpublished doctoral dissertation, Wilmington College, Wilmington, Ohio.

Dwyer, J., & Fischer, D. (1988). Psychometric properties of the coach's version of Leadership Scale for Sports. *Perceptual and Motor Skills, 67,* 795-798.

Gould, D., Tuffey, S., Udry, E., & Loehr, J. (1996a). Burnout in competitive junior tennis players: II. A qualitative analysis. *The Sport Psychologist, 10,* 341-366.

Gould, D., Udry, E., Tuffey, S., & Loehr, J. (1996b). Burnout in competitive junior tennis players: I. A quantitative psychological assessment. *The Sport Psychologist, 10,* 322-340.

Kelley, B. (1994). A model of stress and burnout in collegiate coaches: Effects of gender and time of season. *Research Quarterly for Exercise and Sport, 65,* 48-58.

Kelley, B., Eklund, R., & Ritter-Taylor, M. (1999). Stress and burnout among collegiate tennis coaches. *Journal of Sport and Exercise Psychology, 21,* 113-130.

Lai, C., & Wiggins, S. (2003). Burnout perceptions over time in NCAA division I soccer players. *International Sports Journal, 7,* 120-127.

Maslach, C., & Jackson, S. (1981). The measurement of experienced burnout. *Journal of Occupational Behaviour, 2,* 99-113.

Metzger, M., Kristof, V., & Yoest, D. (2003). The world wide web and the laboratory: A comparison using face recognition. *Cyberpsychology and Behavior: The Impact of the Internet, Multimedia, and Virtual Reality on Behavior and Society, 6,* 613-621.

Meyerson, P., & Tryon, W. (2003). Validating internet research: A test of the psychometric equivalence of Internet and in-person samples. *Behavior Research Methods, Instruments and Computers, 35,* 614-620.

Pastore, D., & Judd, M. (1993). Gender differences in burnout among coaches of women's athletic teams at 2-year colleges. *Sociology of Sport Journal, 10,* 205-212.

Price, M., & Weiss, M. (2000). Relationships among coach burnout, coach behaviors, and athletes' psychological responses. *The Sport Psychologist, 14,* 391-409.

Raedeke, T. (1997). Is athlete burnout more than just stress? A sport commitment perspective. *Journal of Sport and Exercise Psychology, 19,* 396-417.

Raedeke, T., & Smith, A. (2001). Development and preliminary validation of an athlete burnout measure. *Journal of Sport and Exercise Psychology, 23,* 281-306.

Smoll, F., & Smith, R. (1981). Preparation of youth sport coaches: An educational application of sport psychology. *Physical Educator, 38,* 85-94.

Turman, P. (2003). Athletic coaching from an instructional communication perspective: The influence of coach experience on high school wrestlers' preferences and perceptions of coaching behaviors across a season. *Communication Education, 52,* 73-86.

Udry, E., Gould, D., Bridges, D., & Tuffey, S. (1997). People helping people? Examining the social ties of athletes coping with burnout and injury stress. *Journal of Sport and Exercise Psychology, 19,* 368-395.

Vealey, R., Armstrong, L., Comar, W., & Greenleaf, C. (1998). Influence of perceived coaching behaviors on burnout and competitive anxiety in female college athletes. *Journal of Applied Sport Psychology, 10,* 297-318.

Vealey, R., Udry, E., Zimmerman, V., & Soliday, J. (1992). Intrapersonal and situational predictors of coaching burnout. *Journal of Sport and Exercise Psychology, 14,* 40-58.

Weinberg, R., & Gould, D. (2007). *Foundations of sport and exercise psychology.* Champaign, IL: Human Kinetics.

In: Sports and Athletics Developments   ISBN: 978-1-60456-205-7
Editor: James H. Humphrey, pp. 101-110   © 2008 Nova Science Publishers, Inc.

Chapter 6

DEVELOPMENT, CONSTRUCTION, AND VALIDATION OF A SCALE TO MEASURE POSITIVE ILLUSION IN SPORT

*Peter Catina** and Seppo E. Iso-Ahola*

Pennsylvania State University and
University of Maryland

ABSTRACT

The present study was designed to develop a 23-item scale to measure positive illusion in competitive athletes. Positive illusion is a multidimensional psychological construct consisting of the following 3 cognitive characteristics: self-aggrandizement, illusion of control, and unrealistic opitimism. Cronbach's alpha at .84 indicated relatively high internal consistency for the Positive Illusion Sport Scale. Convergent and discriminant validities were assessed by correlating scores from the Scale with scores of self-esteem, hopelessness, optimism, and depression. The Positive Illusion Sport Scale had a moderate positive correlation with self-esteem and optimism and a moderate negative correlation with hopelessness and depression. These findings demonstrate convergent and discriminant validity for the new instrument and suggest that it is psychometrically adequate for research and clinical purposes.

---

* Correspondence to: Dr. Peter Catina, Dept. of Health and Human Development, 1031 Edgecomb Avenue, York, PA 17403. Puc2@psu.edu

Keywords: optimism, motivation, self-esteem, cognitive control.

Positive illusions are common in mentally healthy individuals and may become especially important in the face of threatening information (Taylor, 1983). The term positive illusion represents a multidimensional psychological construct comprised of three sub-constructs. *Self-aggrandizement,* an overly positive self-evaluation, is the perception of one's self, past behavior, and enduring attributes as more positive than is actually the case (Taylor and Armor, 1996). *Illusion of control,* the exaggerated belief in one's personal control, involves the perception that one can bring about primarily positive but not negative outcomes. *Unrealistic optimism,* the perception that the future holds an unrealistically bountiful array of opportunities and a singular absence of adverse events (Taylor, 1989). These cognitive characteristics operate under the overarching framework of positive illusion, which functions as a regulatory mechanism maximizing positive affect and minimizing negative affect.

Positive illusion becomes especially important in the face of threatening social feedback (Taylor, 1983; Taylor and Brown, 1988; 1994; Taylor and Armor, 1996; Taylor and Aspinwall, 1996). According to Taylor (1983), facing negative social feedback may lead to a sense of personal inadequacy, a diminished sense of control, increased feelings of vulnerability, and a sense of despondency and that these negative feelings can be overcome by adopting positive illusions.

The theory of positive illusion has been well established in the literature, but an assessment tool that measures positive illusion has only recently been recognized from am application perspective in sports (Catina and Iso-Ahola, 2004). The implementation of a theory-based instrument assessing the factors that influence levels of success in sport is necessary to understand the role of positive illusion in sport-performance outcomes. Concerning these outcomes, the construct of positive illusion provides a coping strategy for failure through a positive view of the self and an elevated belief in personal control. Although a host of psychological factors examined in the literature such as anxiety, hardiness, locus of control and intrinsic motivation offers insight into explanining sport performance (Iso-Ahola, 1995), positive illusion has not been addressed as a variable influencing favorable outcomes in sport.

A valid and reliable scale will allow investigation of how positive illusions and athletic performance are related. One adaptation to the competitive sports environment may be based on fostering emotional adjustment by instilling a sense of optimism and regaining a perception of control over one's performance. This cognitive coping strategy is a form of creative self-deception. However, it is crucial that the individual demonstrate the ability to maintain augmented views of the self while simultaneously making adaptive use of negative information from the environment (Taylor, 1989). Otherwise, positive illusions run wild and the individual may completely ignore social feedback instead of interpreting it in the best possible light (Taylor and Brown, 1988).

What makes this theory extraordinary is that Taylor and Brown's (1988) formulation of positive illusion seriously challenged a dominant position maintained throughout psychology—that precise contact with reality is a hallmark of mental health. However, their research has shown that accurate perceptions of reality are not essential for mental health. In fact, most people hold inaccurate perceptions of themselves and the world in which they function. Mentally healthy individuals are motivated to avoid psychological distress. A positive sense of self, a need for control, a sense of mastery, and an optimistic view of the future are essential for normal mental functioning (Taylor and Brown, 1988).

Since the athlete's psychological mindset is widely regarded as influencing his or her behavior in sport, more assessment tools are needed in order to broaden the understanding of the mental components that facilitate success in sport. The present study represents an attempt in this regard by outlining the construction of a psychological instrument, establishing its internal consistency, as well as its convergent and discriminant validity by correlating scores from the Positive Illusion Sport Scale with scores of self-esteem, hopelessness, optimism, and depression.

METHOD

An initial pool of 144 items was derived by creating sentences from the theoretical perspectives in the previously cited literature. Critical attention was given to basing the items on the conceptual definitions of the psychological constructs of self-aggrandizement, illusion of control, and unrealistic optimism as provided in the literature. The wording of the sub-constructs of positive illusion, self-aggrandizement (50 items), illusion of control (57 items), and unrealistic optimism (37 items) was designed to capture aspects of these sub-constructs within the context of athletic competition. Content validity was assessed by a panel of 16 athletes registered as sport psychology graduate students who rated the 144 items for relevancy in measuring the sub-constructs of positive illusion using a Likert scale format ranging from -3 (completely irrelevant) to +3 (extremely relevant). Items receiving a rating of 2.00 (relevant) or higher from 70% of the judges were retained and items failing to meet this criterion were deleted; 50 items achieved endorsement and were retained for further analyses.

The majority of the items were not endorsed due to the strict criteria set by the researchers in order to refine the initial item pool. Also, since the items were ultimately designed for athletes, some judges may have failed to separate their own perspective as athletes from their role as judges, even though the instructions attempted to guard against this phenomenon.

The 3 sub-scales (15 items assessing self-aggrandizement, 20 items assessing illusion of control, and 15 items assessing unrealistic optimism) were distributed to 62 competitive collegiate athletes who signed informed consent forms and then indicated the extent to which they agreed with the items on each of the separate sub-scales. A Likert scale format ranging from -3 (strongly disagree) to +3 (strongly agree) was used. The internal consistency of the total 50-item scale was high with an alpha coefficient of .88.

Factor Analysis

A principal component analysis was performed using Promax oblique rotation. Only the first three factors were well defined, but over-extraction of five total factors was used to protect against factor misspecification based on the decelerating decline of eigenvalues in the scree plot. Statistical analysts (Cattell, 1978; Gorsuch, 1983) recommend over-extraction to correctly interpret the information contained in the true factors (Lawrence and Hancock, 1999). Principal components analysis and common factor analysis were used for data reduction. Oblique axis rotation revealed items that loaded on two or more of the primary factors, and/or items with weak loadings below .30; such items were eliminated, reducing the 50 items to the final 23-item instrument. Five of the items were reverse-coded so as to load negatively on the factors (e.g., "I can't do well in sports no matter what I do."). The construct of positive illusion was reflected in three sub-scales: The illusion of control sub-scale was a 9-item scale used to assess exaggerated beliefs of personal control. The self-aggrandizement sub-scale was a 5-item scale designed to assess overly positive self-perceptions, and the unrealistic optimism sub-scale consisted of 9 items measuring unrealistically optimistic views of the future. These measures were combined to form an aggregate score for positive illusion. The correlations among the 3 dimensions were as follows: unrealistic optimism and self-aggrandizement .61, illusion of control and unrealistic optimism .59, illusion of control and self-aggrandizement .45; the overall alpha value was .79.

Assessment of Convergent and Discriminant Validity

To assess the convergent and discriminant validity, the composite score from the Positive Illusion Sport Scale was correlated with scores from the following related constructs: Self-esteem, hopelessness, optimism, and depression. The Positive Illusion Sport Scale was hypothesized to have a moderate positive correlation with the Self-Esteem Scale (Rosenberg, 1965) and the Life Orientation Test (Sheier and Carber, 1985) and to have a moderate negative correlation with Hopelessness (Beck and Steer, 1978) and Depression (Beck, Rial, and Rickels, 1974). These five scales were administered to 139 undergraduate students, 41 of whom were competitive athletes participating in lacrosse, football, soccer, baseball, and gymnastics and 98 were either non-athletic or recreational sport participants. College students from two metropolitan-area campuses comprised the total population.

RESULTS

The resultant three-factor solution accounted for 33.30% of the variance. The 23 items retained had factor loadings of .30 and loaded only on one factor with the majority either approaching or exceeding the .50 level as can be seen in Table 1. By convention, items are retained only if they are equal to or greater than a value of .30 (Bordens and Abbot, 1998). The variances accounted for by factors 1,2, and 3 were 20.4%, 7.0%, and 5.9% respectively.

The final version of the Positive Illusion Sport Scale, representing the three sub-constructs of positive illusion, is presented in Appendix A. Convergent and discriminant validity assessments of the Positive Illusion Sport Scale and the related constructs are presented in Table 2. The internal consistencies for the Self-Esteem, Optimism, Hopelessness, and Depression scales were very high with alpha coefficients of .88, .89, .90, and .90 respectively. Internal consistency for the Positive Illusion Sport Scale was also high at .84.

Correlations among the Positive Illusion Sport Scale and the related constructs are presented in Table 2. As hypothesized, The Positive Illusion Sport Scale showed a moderate positive correlation with self-esteem and optimism and a moderate negative correlation with hopelessness and depression.

Table 1. Factor Loadings for 23 Items Representing Positive Illusion

	Factor I	Factor 2	Factor 3
1. I determine my athletic career.	.76	-	-
3. I can accomplish anything in sport.	.73	-	-
13. My success in sport is due to fate.	.59	-	-
11. Although I try, I can't do well in sports	.58	-	-
8. I can change bad habits easily.	.58	-	-
15. I forget my mistakes and move on.	.40	-	-
19. If I concentrate, I will reach my goals.	.39	-	-
16. I have no control over sport outcomes.	.39	-	-
23. My mind overcomes pain from injury.	.34	-	-
14. I'm better than the average athlete-		.77	-
22. I'm proud of my athletic achievements.	-	.74	-
2. I like to be the center of attention.	-	.52	-
10. I'm an extraordinary athlete.	-	.46	-
17. I always know what to do at contests.	-	.32	-
9. After bad performances, I'll do better.	-		
20. I will be a success in sports.	-	-	.67
21. When setting goals, I expect the best.	-	-	.60
6. I will achieve all my wishes in sport.	-		.46
4. I don't count on good things to happen.	-	-	.45
5. I will always win in sport.	-	-	44
18. I am immune from the dangers in sport.	-	-	44
12. I expect the best in uncertain situations.	-	-	.39
7. It's unrealistic for me to rise to the top.	-		34
Eigenvalues	10.18	3.52	2.95
% of Variance	20.37	7.04	5.90
Cululative %	20.37	27.40	3.30

Table 2. Correlation Matrix for Convergent and Discriminant Validity Assessment of the Positive Illusion Sport Scale and Related Constructs

Scales	M	SD	1	2	3	4	5
1. Positive Illusion	44.60	7.32	.84[1]				
2. Self-esteem	24.25	4.06	.41*	.86[1]			
3. Hopelessness	15.37	6.33	-.37*	-.69*	.86[1]		
4. Optimism	16.35	3.36	.43*	-.66*	-.72*	.83[1]	
5. Depression	5.07	6.49	-.35*	-.49*	.39*	-.41*	.91[1]

[1]AlphaReliability
N=139 (* p<.0001)
Rosenberg Self-EsteemScale
Beck Hopelessness Scale
Life OrientationTest
Beck Depression Inventory

DISCUSSION

These results provide support for the reliability and validity of the Positive Illusion Sport Scale as a measure of positive illusions in competitive athletes. Cronbach's alpha was high and indicated that the 23 items were internally consistent. Further work, however, is needed to establish the test-retest reliability for the Positive Illusion Sport Scale. As for validity, the Positive Illusion Scale correlated in the hypothesized direction and magnitude with the related constructs and measures.

More specifically self-esteem and optimism had a moderate positive correlation with the Positive Illusion Sport Scale, and hopelessness and depression had a moderate negative correlation with the Scale. These findings demonstrate considerable convergent and discriminant validity for the new instrument and suggest that it is psychometrically adequate for research purposes. More research is needed to further validate the measure, especially it if is to be used for teaching and cultivating positive illusion in athletes who may have low levels in this cognitive dimension.

Besides the demonstrated convergent and discriminant validity, the Positive Illusion Sport Scale has predictive validity as well. Further sequencing of these statistical procedures has been justified by the successful demonstration of the utility of the scale in a sport performance framework (Catina and Iso-Ahola, 2004). Given that no other scales of positive illusion exist, cultivating this new measure is necessary to to further assess its utility across a broader range of sport contexts.

The Positive Illusion Sport Scale evolved from empirical thrust specifically intended to create a scale with unique structural and construct validity qualities. Conceptually, the scale is based on the well-established theory of positive illusion, which may have a high degree of relevance to researchers interested in understanding more about the role of this cognitive construct in human performance in general and athletic performance in particular.

APPENDIX :
POSITIVE ILLUSION SPORT SCALE

Directions

Below are some sentences that describe certain feelings that different athletes have. Read each item carefully and think about your sport. You will probably agree with some items and disagree with others. We are interested in the extent to which you agree or disagree with each of the items.

Indicate the extent to which you agree or disagree by circling the appropriate number following each sentence. The numbers and their meanings are indicated below:

If you disagree strongly: circle -3
If you disagree: circle -2
If you disagree slightly: circle –1

If you agree slightly: circle +1
If you agree: circle +2
If you agree strongly: circle +3

Be as honest and accurate as you can with your responses. Thank you.

	Disagree Strongly	Disagree	Disagree Slightly	Agree Slightly	Agree	Agree Strongly
1. My own action.is determined mostly by my own actions	-3	-2	-1	+1	+2	
	+3					
2. I really like to be the center of attention during my sport event.	-3	-2	-1	+1	+2	+3
3. If I put my mind to it, I can accomplish just about about anything in sport.	-3	-2	-1	+1	+2	+3
4..I rarely count on good things to happen to me while competing in sport.	-3	-2	-1	+1	+2	
5.I will stay on top no matter how tough the competition gets.	-3	-2	-1	+1	+2	+3
6. I will achieve the things I wish for.	-3	-2	-1	+1	+2	+3
7. I believe that it is unrealistic to think that someday I will rise to the top level of my sport.	-3	-2	-1	+1	+2	+3

	Disagree Strongly	Disagree	Disagree Slightly	Agree Slightly	Agree	Agree Strongly
8. I can change old habits that I may have developed in my sport technique without much difficulty and without slipping back.	-3	-2	-1	+1	+2	+3
9. After a bad performance, I am usually certain that I will do better next time.	-3	-2	-1	+1	+2	+3
10 I am an extraordinary athlete.	-3	-2	-1	+1	+2	+3
11. I can't do well in sports no matter what I do.	-3	-2	-1	+1	+2	+3
12. In uncertain situations in sport, I usually expect the best.	-3	-2	-1	+1	+2	+3
13. My success in sport has largely been a matter of being in the right place at the right time.	-3	-2	-1	+1	+2	+3
14. I am more capable of succeeding in sports than the average athlete is.	-3	-2	-1	+1	+2	+3
15. If I make an awkward mistake in competition, I can soon forget it and concentrate on the next sport task.	-3	-2	-1	+1	+2	+3
16. I have no control over the outcomes associated with my sport.	-3	-2	-1	+1	+2	+3
17 I always know what I am going to during competition.	-3	-2	-1	+1	+2	+3
18 With regard to the dangers associated with competing in my sport, I expect others to be the victims of misfortune rather than myself.	-3	-2	-1	+1	+2	+3
19 If I concentrate on the goals that I have set for competition, I will achieve them.	-3	-2	-1	+1	+2	+3
20. I will be a success in sports.	-3	-2	-1	+1	+2	+3
21 When setting my performance goals, I am usually happy at heart because I expect success.	-3	-2	-1	+1	+3	
22. I am proud of my athletic accomp	-3	-2	-1	+1	+2	+3
23. If I had a nagging injury, it would not prevent me from competing because my mind can overcome the pain.	-3	-2	-1	+1	+2	+3

REFERENCES

Beck, A.T., Rial, W.Y., and Rickels, K. (1974). Beck Depression Inventory (rev.ed.). Short form of depression inventory: Cross-validation. *Psychological Reports,* 34, 1184-1186.

Beck, A.T., and Steer, R.A. (1978). *Beck Hopelessness Scale* (rev.ed.). University of Pennsylvania, Philadelphia, PA: Center for Cognitive Therapy.

Bordens, K.S., and Abbot, B.B. (1998). *Research design and methods: A process approach (3ʳᵈ ed.).* Mountain View, CA: Mayfield.

Catina, P.D., and Iso-Ahola, S.E. (2004). Positive illusion and athletic success. *International Sports Journal,* 8, 80-93.

Cattell, R.B. (1978). *The scientific use of factoral analysis in behavioral and life sciences.* New York: Plenum.

Gorsuch, R.L. (1983). *Factor analysis.* Hillsdale, NJ: Lawrence Erlbaum.

Rosenberg, M. (1965). *Society and the adolescent self-image.* Princeton, NJ: Princeton University Press.

Iso-Ahola, S.E. (1995). Intrapersonal and interpersonal factors in athletic performance. *Scandinavian Journal of Medicine and Science in Sports,* 5, 191-199.

Sheier, M.F., and Carver, C.S. (1985). Optimism, coping and health: Assessment and Implications of generalized outcome expectancies. *Health Psychology,* 4, 219-247.

Taylor, S.E. (1983). Adjustment to threatening events. *American Psychologist,* 38, 1161-1173.

Taylor, S.E. (1989). *Positive illusions: Creative self-deception and the healthy mind.* New York. Basic Books, Inc.

Taylor, S.E., and Armor, D.A. (1996). Positive illusions and coping with adversity. *Journal of Personality,* 64, 873-898.

Taylor, S.E., and Aspinwall, L.G. (1996). Mediating and moderating processes in psychological stress: Appraisal, coping, resistance, and vulnerability. In H.B. Kaplan (Ed.), *Psychological stress: Perspectives on structure, theory, life-course, and methods* (pp. 71-100). San Diego: Academic Press.

Taylor, S.E., and Brown, J.D. (1988). Illusion and well-being: A social psychological perspective on mental health. *Psychological bulletin,* 103, 193-210.

Taylor, S.E. and Brown, J.D. (1994). Positive illusions and well-being revisited: Separating fact from fiction. *Psychological Bulletin,* 116, 1, 21-27.

Taylor, S.E., and Gollwitzer, P.M. (1995). Effects of mindset on positive illusions. *Journal of Personality and Social Psychology,* 69, 213-226.

INDEX

J

L

M

T

U

V

validity, ix, 7, 10, 11, 12, 16, 19, 34, 48, 52,
86, 87, 101, 103, 105, 107
values, 8, 17, 49, 52, 54
variable(s), 4, 6, 7, 8, 10, 11, 12, 13, 16, 17,
18, 19, 21, 22, 30, 33, 39, 48, 49, 56, 86,
87, 90, 91, 92, 93, 94, 98, 102
variance, viii, 8, 35, 45, 48, 52, 92, 105
venue, 55
victims, 109
video games, 6
Virginia, 81
voice, 64
volleyball, 60
vulnerability, 102, 110

W

warrants, 39
Washington, 24
web, 65, 88, 100
webpages, 54
well-being, 30, 31, 44, 110
winning, 31
women, viii, 36, 44, 45, 46, 47, 52, 53, 54, 55,
56, 59, 60, 62, 63, 65, 72, 77, 78, 100
World War II, 2